# Low-Water Veggie Gardening: How to Make a Drought-Resistant Vegetable Garden, Conserve Water, and Grow Your Own Food

ALINA NIEMI

Alina's Pencil Publishing

2014

# DEDICATION

For Mary Meeker, who thought she could no longer garden because of drought.

Aunty Mary, I hope this will help change your mind.
## HaPPY GRoWiNG!

Find updates and corrections at www.alinaspencil.com

For more information, please contact the publisher at www.alinaspencil.com

ISBN: 978-1-937371-09-8

# Contents

Why Bother? ........................................................................ 1

  What this book will not teach you: ........................... 1

  What this book will teach you: ................................... 1

  Why should you grow your own vegetables? ............ 4

    It's cheaper ................................................................ 5

    You have control ....................................................... 5

    It's sustainable ......................................................... 7

    What's old is new again .......................................... 8

    Control your situation ............................................. 9

    Global warming......................................................... 9

    Crazy weather ......................................................... 10

    Seed saving .............................................................. 11

    Open-pollinated seeds ........................................... 12

    In the event of a disaster ....................................... 13

  It's healthier for you and the environment ............ 14

    Reduces water runoff ............................................. 14

    A mini-ecosystem ................................................... 14

    Control the safety of your food ............................. 14

    Less energy for transportation.............................. 18

    Fresher food, more nutrients ................................ 18

  Additional Benefits ..................................................... 18

    Connection to nature .............................................. 18

A plethora of choices ...................................................... 20

Great to get kids involved ............................................. 22

## How Does Nature Do It? ............................................. 24

Growth in a forest ........................................................ 24

Life in a desert ............................................................. 24

The basic principles ..................................................... 25

Everything is recycled .............................................. 25

There is minimal input .............................................. 25

Plants have adapted to local conditions ................... 26

Water is used effectively ........................................... 26

There is great biodiversity ........................................ 27

## Real-World Proof ...................................................... 29

China ........................................................................... 29

Saudi Arabia ............................................................... 31

Ethiopia ...................................................................... 32

Change is possible ....................................................... 33

## The Big Picture ......................................................... 34

What happens to water? .............................................. 34

What happens to plants? ............................................. 35

The solution for gardening in a drought..................... 36

Permaculture and Natural Farming............................. 37

## The Dirt on Dirt ....................................................... 39

Soil structure and composition ................................... 39

It's a living ecosystem ................................................. 40

We are not humans .................................................. 41

Be like the forest.................................................... 43

Compost, aka "Black Gold" .................................... 43

Composting in a nutshell .................................... 44

What's free and fabulous? ...................................... 46

Wriggle while you work......................................... 48

Your throne of fertility .......................................... 48

You scratch my roots, I'll scratch yours.................. 49

Work less and get better results............................. 50

Stop Spouting Off: How to Reduce Evaporation and Runoff
.................................................................................52

Transpiration........................................................... 52

Why water is lost ................................................. 53

Rolling, rolling, rolling: How to reduce runoff ..... 59

The Fountain of Life: Water and How to Save It ................. 62

Water conservation ................................................ 62

Stop leaks............................................................. 62

Turn off the tap.................................................... 62

Use water-wise shower faucets ............................ 63

Re-use your water ............................................... 63

Your dirty water ................................................. 64

Rain is nature's gold: How to collect it................. 65

Low-tech high tech: Fog collectors...................... 67

Watering your plants .............................................. 69

Put it where it counts...........................................................69

Water deeply ......................................................................75

When to water for the most benefit ................................75

How much to water? ........................................................76

Seed starting ideas............................................................78

It's Not What You Do, It's How You Do It:  Water-Saving
Garden Types...................................................................83

Not just for breakfast .....................................................83

Square foot gardening .....................................................84

Lasagna gardening:  In-place layering .......................85

Subversive designs:  Sub-irrigated planters.........................85

Go shopping for grow bags .........................................91

The ghetto gardens .......................................................93

Aquaponics and Pee-ponics .......................................95

Don't throw it out:  Bottle tower and PVC pipe gardens....95

The pizza and pie combo.................................................97

Going in circles:  Spiral garden.....................................99

Go Big if You Can:  Modifying Your Landscape ................. 102

Bury the evidence ..........................................................103

Water Engineering...........................................................105

Basic principles ..............................................................106

Swales.............................................................................107

Gabions..........................................................................111

Planting:  The What, Where, How and Why....................... 113

What to plant..................................................................113

    Choosing what to grow.........................................113

    Seeds or seedlings?................................................117

    Open-pollinated or heirlooms.............................119

    Drought-resistant versus drought-tolerant........119

    Drought-resistant or normal?...............................120

    Drought- and heat-tolerant varieties..................121

Garden buddies: Companion planting for a harmonious garden..................................................................................125

    The three sisters.....................................................128

    Beneficial attractors..............................................129

    Tips for healthy seedlings.....................................130

    Where to plant........................................................130

    When to plant.........................................................131

    How to plant...........................................................132

    Tips for pepper and tomato seedlings.................132

    Air pruning.............................................................133

General Gardening Tips.............................................. 134

    Pest control.............................................................134

    Gardening on a budget..........................................135

    Reuse materials whenever possible.....................135

    Be careful of free stuff..........................................135

    Reuse discarded toilet tanks................................136

    Free seeds...............................................................137

Keep seeds dry and cool ...................................................... 138

Find sources for more organic materials ........................... 138

Start new plants from old ................................................... 138

What to do with your harvest .............................................. 138

Food preservation methods ............................................... 139

Donate .................................................................................. 139

Sell ........................................................................................ 139

Learn More: Resources ................................................ 140

In person .............................................................................. 140

Take a walk ........................................................................... 140

Community gardens ............................................................ 140

Board of Water Supply ....................................................... 141

Local nurseries and garden centers ................................. 141

University Extension Offices ............................................. 141

Online .................................................................................... 142

Gardening forums ............................................................... 142

Sources for Seeds ............................................................... 143

Links to more information online ..................................... 145

Bibliography ..................................................................... 151

Index ................................................................................. 155

Can you help me? ............................................................ 177

Also by the author: ............................................................. 178

# ACKNOWLEDGMENTS

This book would never have been possible without the input from countless individuals all over the world. Thanks to their innovation, sweat, labor, and willingness to share the results of their experience, we can all learn and improve.

I'm grateful to all the backyard farmers, market gardeners, visionaries, and others who believe it's worth the time and trouble to experiment and learn about sustainable agriculture. Without the willingness to take chances, put in the required years of effort, and then make videos, write books, and post on online forums, we would all be alone, making the same mistakes over and over. By sharing our knowledge with others, we can make lasting change for the better health of the people, animals, and organisms living on earth, and indeed, for the better health of our precious planet itself.

Nature has miraculous powers of rejuvenation that we can tap into if we are willing to be conscientious students. I wish you much success and joy in your gardening adventures!

# CHAPTER 1
## Why Bother?

### What this book will not teach you:

- What varieties to plant
- Specific garden designs or layouts
- How to grow in an arid region without watering your plants (also known as dry farming)
- Basic vegetable gardening

### What this book will teach you:

- How to conserve water
- How to make the best use of any moisture in your environment, including rain, fog, or mist
- How others have grown food with and without irrigation
- What varieties others have found drought-resistant
- How to choose the best plants for your area
- How to grow vegetables using as little water as possible
- Sustainable methods to increase soil fertility and moisture-holding properties
- Several types of productive, water-wise gardens

It was very ironic that soon after I started writing this book, our area was blanketed in rains. Tropical storms and hurricanes often plague us in Hawaii, so the weather is always unpredictable and constantly changing. While we have typically sunny, warm days and light showers, especially in the mountains and valleys, the rest of the islands can have snow (on the volcano tops), desert, and long periods without rain.

Meanwhile, my aunty in California was bemoaning the fact that a long, hard drought meant she could no longer garden. But I knew that was not the case. She did not need to abandon gardening altogether. In fact, I knew she could get higher yields and more productivity, using very little water, simply by choosing efficient gardening methods and sustainable principles. But when I looked for a book to point her to, there was nothing available.

Sure, there were books on organic gardening. More than you can shake a trowel at. A few on drought-tolerant garden design. But most of those covered landscape planting, trees, shrubs, and flowers, with almost no information on vegetable gardening.

So this book was born. I have used some of the methods already in my gardening over the last 20+ years. I learn more every day and keep experimenting, to get the most water-efficient, productive vegetable garden I can.

On the whole, vegetables require more water than flowers, shrubs, and trees. But there are many ways you can make efficient use of the water you give your vegetables. And there are many ways to get more moisture. Most of them go untapped by the average gardener (pun intended).

The recent crazy climate changes have meant that areas of the world that never get rain are getting storms, parts that are hot are getting snowed on, and areas that are used to rain and cold are dry and hot. So even those of us in areas that normally get a generous amount of rain need to know what to do in times of drought, because nothing about the weather is predictable any more.

I walked around Tokyo during a flight layover in October, sweating in the almost 80-degree sunshine, when in the past, fall temperatures were well below that. I certainly did not need the fleece jacket that I had in my carry-on bag.

Drought is plaguing much of the world right now, including western and central states of the U.S., such as Oregon, California, and Nevada. Over 80% of the state of Queensland, Australia, the largest area in the state's history, has been declared in drought.

Areas of the world that rely on moisture from a rainy season have gotten less than normal, or none whatsoever in recent years. There is even a Global Drought Information System website at www.drought.gov.

Many places are experiencing abnormal weather. Yet everyone needs to eat. With some conventional, commercial farmers not even bothering to plant crops, because of predictions of continuing water shortages, the availability of food is sure to become an issue. Even if food continues to be available, prices are on the rise and show no signs of stopping.

People everywhere are wondering how they can take steps to either begin a food garden, or continue to grow their vegetables in drought conditions. This book will give you lots of ideas, inspiration, and hope. All over the world, projects and individuals are taking steps to provide food, while reducing the need for resources such as water, electricity, and materials.

Our over-reliance on traditional farming methods and energy production has worked okay so far, but everything is changing. We cannot continue to do things the way we have been, because our environment doesn't work the way it has in the past.

You cannot continue to sprinkler-water your lawn or garden when mandatory water restrictions are in place. How is it possible to use even less water than you would for grass, and get more food than you can consume? Read about how people all over the world are doing just that, in this book.

The first part of this book discusses the arguments: Why bother growing your own food? Why consider organic methods? What do human activities have to do with fertility and climate change? And does any of this stuff really work?

The second part will show you the principles and methods: How to conserve water, how to irrigate your crops, how to mimic nature to build healthy soil, how to choose the best plants for your area and weather, and how to learn more.

Take these ideas and principles. Play with them. Try them. Adapt them. Tinker with them. Try something else. Connect with like-minded others and come up with new things to experiment with.

Gardening is like anything else in life. It takes work, patience, and dedication in order to see results. You do not plant a seed on Sunday and eat from it on Thursday. If you stop tending to your garden, it will stop providing for you.

But you will learn that there are ways to make growing your own vegetables as easy and efficient as possible. And you will see results. So roll up your sleeves and get digging.

Well, not right away. Read first, and take action later. Because having a plan based on solid principles can mean the difference between food or famine, fruitfulness or failure.

## Why should you grow your own vegetables?

It's so easy nowadays to run to the grocery store or warehouse club and fill up with cheap produce all year long. Why bother with growing your own, hauling bags of stinky manure, straining your back, digging trenches, weeding, watering, hunting down bugs and slugs, moles and voles, deer and rabbits and raccoons?

Besides, if you live in a part of the country where you are affected by drought, you may be under water restrictions or rationing, and don't want to waste any of that on plants that may or may not grow. So why bother with all this?

## It's cheaper

Have you noticed the price of food lately? You may be in sticker shock now, but the recent wild, unpredictable weather is sure to result in even higher food prices in the future. Why?

Crop failures, the loss of pollinating bees, drought, snow in Georgia, and floods means less available food. Yet there are just as many people who have to eat. What does that mean for prices? They skyrocket.

Costs for fuel, for heavy machinery to do the work and transportation, chemical fertilizers and pesticides, warehouse and refrigeration space, packaging, and labor are all factored into the price consumers pay at the store or market. So are any extras, such as using heaters to warm your citrus trees when the weather gets too cold, as California farmers did.

One packet of vegetable seeds, containing anywhere from 10 to 300 seeds, costs about $2.00 to $3.00. Even if you had to plant the entire packet to get one plant, that is still cheaper than what you would pay for harvested produce at retail prices.

Yes, there are added costs in gardening, such as tools, equipment, soil amendments, and containers. But you can successfully garden on a shoestring budget and more than recoup your costs in one season.

## You have control

### Choose your favorites

When you grow your own food, you grow what you like to eat. You are not limited by what is offered at the store, or by the price you have to pay.

Do you love kale? Organic kale can get pricey. The local health food store sells a bunch, containing about 5 leaves, for $7.00. I can pick that easily from one or two plants. Those plants will continue to produce that much for me, for several months, at very little added cost.

## GMOs

Companies have used genetic engineering to create new vegetables and fruits that have miraculous powers not otherwise found in nature. For example, tomatoes that will not get ripe for weeks on end, so they can be picked green and stored in warehouses, then shipped all over the world, without rotting or getting smashed.

Or corn that has insecticides already inside the plants, so that when bugs eat the corn, they die.

That is the theory, anyway. In reality, these crops have already wreaked havoc on neighboring farms, because they spread beyond the boundaries of the farms where the crops are grown. Farmers on adjoining land have suffered reduced yields and crop failure, and it seems there is nothing they can do about it.

GMOs (Genetically Modified Organisms) are not currently regulated in the United States. That's why there is no mention of them on food labels. But the vast majority of corn and soybeans in the U.S. is already genetically modified. It's in the food you eat, and being sold in stores. You just don't know it.

Scientists do not even know the long-term effects of GMOs on our bodies or the environment. There is a possibility they are horrendously destructive, yet we may not find this out for decades to come.

You, the consumer, get to be the guinea pig in a living laboratory. Who stands to benefit from using GMOs? The companies who manufacture those seeds. They stand to make a lot of money by selling them. And if, sometime down the line, we find out they are harmful? Oh well, they'll stop making them.

You may think the entire GMO debate is a waste of time. You may have nothing against them and think this is nothing but a rant by some tree-hugging, air-head hippie.

Fine. Let's assume GMOs cause zero damage and are perfectly healthy. You can buy seeds from anywhere and not care if those seeds have had any genetic modification.

But if you *do* care, you have the option to choose to buy seeds that are organically grown. Organic foods cannot contain any GMOs.

Also, many seed growers test their seeds for GMOs and will not sell any that have them. So you can decide for yourself, and choose to purchase seeds from vendors who feel the same way you do, and avoid growing GMO produce.

## It's sustainable

### What the heck is sustainability, anyway?

Simply put, sustainability is the ability of something to endure. I don't mean once you plant your vegetables, they will be there forever. (Although there are perennial plants you can put in your garden that will provide food for you for years to come, this book will cover mostly annual vegetable crops, because that's what most people grow.)

But I do mean your gardening system can endure. If the materials you use are organic materials, from the land and living organisms, they will break down into nutrients that feed your garden.

Rather than kill the microorganisms in your soil by using sterile growing mediums and adding synthetic chemicals, you can create an ever-improving mini-ecosystem. You may start out with next to nothing in the way of soil and productivity, but there are ways to start producing food with almost nothing. Then you return everything back to the soil, creating a never-ending cycle of life and death and life again. Over time, you will see increased yields and productivity and a more fertile, healthier land.

Unlike conventional or subsistence farming, which relies on mono-cropping (growing large swaths of one crop, such as corn or soybeans), tilling, and chemical additions, plus large amounts of water, fertilizers, and pesticides, you will let nature do the work for you, as it knows how to do. There will be challenges, certainly--don't think these methods of gardening are picture perfect. But your garden and plants will increasingly be able to deal with climate change, drought, and the unexpected, and continue to produce abundantly.

## What's old is new again

When I was in school in the 1970s, bell bottom pants, platform shoes, and psychedelic prints were in fashion. Well, platform shoes are on the way out (again), and psychedelic prints are on the way in. Groovy! If I had kept my wardrobe, I could be making a fortune selling it online!

What's old is fashionable again, but it's not just about looks. With gardening and sustainability, caring for the environment is no longer a hippies-only pastime. Backyard gardening, homesteading, and urban poultry-raising are all on the rise, not because they are fads, but because they make sense.

During World Wars I and II, people were encouraged to grow Victory Gardens in their yards, to help provide food that was in short supply. The gardens were fabulously successful, producing 40% of the vegetables consumed in the U.S. during World War II.

Today, having a garden in your yard is popular once again, but they are being called "Kitchen Gardens" and "Urban Gardens" instead. And this is a trend that is growing, fueled by people's desires, not by government's encouragement.

People are taking their power back. They want safe, reliable food sources, without wondering what something is made of. They are tired of finding out after the fact that something they are eating is loaded with unhealthy chemicals, or farmed using harmful or questionable practices.

## Control your situation

Any time you go to a store to buy your food, you are dependent on the growers, distributors, and retailers that provide it. When you buy hybrid seeds from a company, you need to get new seeds from them every year.

But if you grow your own food, you can save seeds from open-pollinated or heirloom plants. This puts the power back in your hands. You have the ability to feed yourself season after season, regardless of the whims of any companies, growers, or stores.

## Global warming

Global warming is the gradual, increasing temperature all over the world, caused by a blanket of gases in the atmosphere. The theory is that the normal climate cycles have been thrown out of whack due to destroying large sections of natural vegetation, such as woodlands, rainforest or jungle. Plants that would normally filter toxins and carbon dioxide from the air are no longer there, so they don't cool the earth and cause rainfall. Instead, the gases remain in the air.

Eating meat has also caused more gases. Those cows, pigs, and chickens all produce toxic gases in their feces, and woods, prairies, and forests have been cleared and destroyed in order to raise these animals to feed us. Overgrazing by domestic animals in some areas has left the land barren and unable to support any life whatsoever. (See Real World Proof, Chapter 3).

In addition, a larger human population burns wood for fuel, spewing gases into the air. There were 7 billion people on earth in 2010. That is double what existed only 50 years ago. People use vehicles that spew toxic fumes into the atmosphere every time they drive somewhere. Commercial agriculture also relies on petroleum-fueled machinery.

This high amount of chemical pollutants, called "greenhouse gases," forms a blanket over the earth, causing higher temperatures. If you sit in a car on a hot day, with the windows closed, you will overheat and eventually die. In the same way, those gases are like the car, trapping heat, and you are like the planet. You are stuck inside, with the temperature rising.

Rising temperatures heat water, too, which covers 71% of the planet, causing far-reaching effects. Warmer ocean waters cause melting of glacier ice, which raises the water level. Low-lying communities get flooded, and people are forced to move to higher ground.

Warmer ocean waters also change the balance we've had for centuries by killing off some species and allowing others to flourish. This can cause dangerously low levels of some species of fish and seafood, meaning we have less food.

## Crazy weather

How do you like the recent crazy weather we've been having? Floods, droughts, snow storms, hurricanes, are all affected by the water cycle and how much water and wind are in the atmosphere. Less rain means wildfires spread out of control, like they did in Colorado, Arizona, and Oregon in 2002. Dust storms have plagued Montana and Kansas, and floods have damaged parts of Texas and North Dakota.

Everything is connected on the earth. What we do in one part of the world matters to people in other parts, and vice versa. There are lines of separation on a map, but not in the air, water, or on land. Nature does not distinguish between countries and cultures. The polluted air over China eventually blows to other countries, including the U.S.

Ocean water in California and Japan are the same water, that of the Pacific Ocean. Radiation contamination from a nuclear disaster in Fukushima, Japan, has already made its way to the U.S. According to a report by the National Academy of Sciences, Pacific Bluefin tuna carried Fukushima-derived radionuclides across the entire North Pacific Ocean.[1]

The theory is that people have caused this climate change. You may not believe that what people do on the planet has anything whatsoever to do with rising temperatures or crazy, abnormal weather. Fair enough.

But just maybe the reduction in plants worldwide has contributed to these changing weather patterns. And maybe by changing our environment and landscape, and growing plants in areas that have been barren, dry, desserts, barely able to grow anything, we can reverse the trend and move back toward what used to be normal weather.

For now, though, let's just assume global warming is here to stay, and that the earth's temperatures will continue to rise, and that we will continue to have crazy weather. Growing your own vegetables allows you to adapt to changing weather conditions. While commercial farmers struggle to deal with heat and drought, you can apply some of the principles covered in this book, and still have food to eat, while conserving money and water at the same time.

## Seed saving

When you grow your own vegetables, you can save seeds from some of what you plant, then use them for a future crop. This

---

[1] Steve Elwart, "Japan Radiation Poisoning America?" *WND Health*, December 30, 2013, http://www.wnd.com/2013/12/japan-radiation-poisoning-america/ (accessed April 24, 2014).

allows you to be more self-sufficient. You do not need to rely on a seed company to provide you with seed in order to grow something.

You don't need to grow only the varieties offered by seed companies, either. Many families have passed down seeds from generation to generation. Called heirloom seeds, they have stood the test of time, adapting to growing conditions in one, and often, several, areas, as a family moves from place to place.

## Open-pollinated seeds

Seeds that will produce offspring with the same characteristics as the parent plant are open-pollinated seeds. They are different from hybrid seeds, which are developed by seed companies to produce plants with certain characteristics, such as slower ripening, or resistance to weather conditions or diseases.

Hybrid seeds often will not produce offspring that are fertile, or they may not have the same qualities that parent plants had. In other words, you may be able to grow another plant from seeds you have saved from a hybrid plant, but seeds saved from that second generation will not produce any more plants.

Or you might save hybrid tomato seeds, only to find that the plant you get from those seeds is entirely different from its parent plant. Instead of plump, disease-resistant cherry tomatoes, you end up with a sprawling, sickly vine of tiny, berry-like fruits. That means you need to go back to the seed company and buy more seeds. Great luck for the seed company, eh?

Any time you choose to plant open-pollinated (or heirloom) seeds, you keep the power in your hands, not in the seed companies. And yes, you guessed it right. Many of those seed companies are the same ones that produce genetically-modified seeds, GMOs. Are you seeing any patterns here?

## In the event of a disaster

Some people are certain that in the coming decades, within their lifetimes or that of their children, they will experience a horrible disaster that leaves people homeless. They may end up in a situation where communication is shut down, electricity, gas, and running water are unavailable, and food is scarce or unavailable.

Perhaps it will be a flood, storm, earthquake, or other natural disaster. Maybe it will be war or uprising. It might even be something like a solar flare or an asteroid colliding with earth.

In these situations, you can use your own food stash, survival skills, and other knowledge, to fare better than others around you. If you had a garden, you'd already be ahead of the vast majority of people in your community. Assuming your garden survives damage, that is.

But even if your garden gets destroyed, you will have the knowledge and skills to begin to grow for yourself, just like generations of people before you have done, as they moved from one part of the country to another, or emigrated from one country to this one.

Most of us have ancestors who moved to the United States from other countries. And you can bet many of them had seeds from their favorite crops, which they planted and grew in their new homes.

Growing your own food helps provide a measure of food stability and security, the ability to get food no matter what happens in the world around you. We all need to eat in order to survive. Gardening can give you that extra edge. And if there is no disaster? Lucky you! You'll still be smacking your lips!

# It's healthier for you and the environment

## Reduces water runoff

When land is denuded and barren, it no longer has the capacity to hold water. When it rains, the water washes soil away with it, causing mudslides, flood, and more erosion. The dirty water ends up in rivers, streams, and oceans, causing pollution and further problems.

But if that same land had plants on it, these problems would not occur, or they would be reduced. The plant roots would hold moisture in the soil, allowing it to stay in place.

## A mini-ecosystem

Plant leaves and branches help to convert carbon dioxide in the air into oxygen, which we breathe. They trap moisture and create a mini-ecosystem which attracts insects, birds, butterflies, and other creatures, adding to the planet's biodiversity. They filter toxins out of the air and water, and the soil creates a natural filter for rain, which slowly seeps into the earth far below, often ending up as our future drinking water.

When you grow your own garden, you can control and create that ecosystem. You have the power to choose what to put into it, and what to leave out. You can fill it with hybrid plants, synthetic fertilizers, and chemical pest- and disease-killers. Or you can use open-pollinated or heirloom plants, natural soil amendments, and nature's own checks and balances.

## Control the safety of your food

### Reduce your exposure to toxic chemicals

The Environmental Protection Agency (EPA) is the controlling force behind what kind of toxic chemicals are allowed on food crops in the United States. The EPA sets limits on how much of a pesticide may be used on food during growing and processing, and how much can remain on the food you buy.

These levels for toxic pesticide residue, called tolerances, are different for each pesticide being used. However, -- and this is a very important point--, they do not set a limit on the **number** of pesticides allowed.

So you can have a level of Pesticide A that is at an allowable amount, plus Pesticide B at an allowed level, plus Pesticides C, D, E, F, G, and H. It might scare you to know there are tolerances for 9,700 different chemicals set by the agency.

9,700 chemicals! That means you can have any combination of those 9,700 chemicals on any food you eat.

The tolerances are set based on what the agency believes to be a reasonable amount, considering the safety of people in mind. And there are even more chemicals with no limits whatsoever, because the EPA considers them safe for human consumption.

Their definition of pesticide:

> The term pesticide includes many kinds of ingredients used in products, such as insecticides, fungicides, rodenticides, insect repellants, weed killers, antimicrobials, and swimming pool chemicals, which are designed to prevent, destroy, repel, or reduce pests of any sort.[2]

Not only are there no limits to the number of pesticides allowed, but there are also no studies conducted on the hazards or toxicity of any combination of those 9,700 chemicals. I think it is reasonable to assume that there must be combinations of pesticides, all of which are intended to kill something, that can

---

[2] U. S. Environmental Protection Agency, *U. S. Environmental Protection Agency*, http://www.epa.gov/pesticides/factsheets/stprf.htm (accessed April 24, 2014).

cause harm to humans. We just have no data to support this assumption.

I don't know about you, but the thought of consuming 9,700 toxic chemicals (they are intended to kill something, after all) is scary. The thought of consuming even *one* of them is scary. It's impossible to avoid toxins altogether, but I prefer to limit my exposure to them as much as I can.

When you grow your own food, you know exactly what chemicals have or have not been used. When you apply a pesticide, you are making a conscious choice that you will likely ingest some lingering residue when you eat your produce later.

But when you purchase something that someone else grew, you have no idea what they have or have not applied. Even if the label states that something was "organic" or "organically grown," you can only assume that the farmer followed the standard practices set by the USDA, the United States Department of Agriculture, the agency that regulates certification, production, handling, and labeling of USDA organic products. You really have no way to be sure.

Even in organic farming, some synthetic chemicals are allowed for pest or disease control when other safer, more natural methods, such as mulching, crop rotation, and applying plant or animal material, have not worked. You still have no way of knowing which of those chemicals, if any, were used, if you did not grow the food yourself.

But if you grow your own crops, you can decide to use as few of those toxic chemicals as possible, which means you ingest fewer of them. It is absolutely possible to grow vegetables and rarely need to spray anything more dangerous than some soapy water or baking soda solution. I've done it for more than 20 years. That certainly sounds safer than a potential chemical cocktail of up to 9,700 toxins!

## Food recalls

In October, 2013, 22,849 pounds of broccoli salad kit products were recalled due to concerns about possible *Listeria monocytogenes* contamination in the salad dressing. According to the U.S. Department of Agriculture's Food Safety and Inspection Service (FSIS):

> *L. monocytogenes can cause fever, muscle aches, headache, stiff neck, confusion, loss of balance and convulsions sometimes preceded by diarrhea or other gastrointestinal symptoms. An invasive infection spreads beyond the gastrointestinal tract. In pregnant women, the infection can cause miscarriages, stillbirths, premature delivery or life-threatening infection of the newborn. In addition, serious and sometimes fatal infections in older adults and persons with weakened immune systems.*[3]

While the vast majority of food recalls contain animal products, such as meat and poultry, there have been some recalls of produce. Often these problems are traced to contamination of water supplies or equipment by animal excrement. Still, they can affect you, the consumer.

The only way you can avoid them is by growing your own food and using safe practices and hygiene if you handle manures of any kind, including as fertilizer in an organic garden. Getting sick from your own home-grown produce is rare.

---

[3] Food Safety and Inspection Service, U. S. Department of Agriculture, *Recalls and Public Health Alerts*, http://www.fsis.usda.gov/wps/wcm/connect/FSIS-Content/internet/main/topics/recalls-and-public-health-alerts/recall-case-archive/archive/2013/recall-062-2013-expansion (accessed April 24, 2014).

## Less energy for transportation

Most food is grown on a farm or nursery, transported to a factory to be processed, then to a distributor, then to a retailer, where you buy it and transport it home. In the process, many gallons of fuel are used for moving the goods. Even more is used for refrigeration and storage.

Growing your own food considerably reduces the amount of fuel needed. Sometimes you can pick from your garden and walk a few yards, into your kitchen, and eat it. No polluting fuels required!

## Fresher food, more nutrients

Anyone who has grown tomatoes in their garden can tell you that the taste and aroma cannot even be compared to what you buy in a store. "Cardboard," "mealy," and "gross" have been used to describe store-bought tomatoes. "Heavenly," "tastes like when I was a kid," and "tangy with just a hint of sweet to round it out" have described home-grown ones. Which would you rather eat?

You can pick food from your garden and eat it in a matter of seconds. The best you can hope for when you buy something at a market is less than 24 hours later than it was picked. The sooner you eat your produce after it is picked, the more nutrients are retained. A fresh sugar snap pea or perfectly ripe strawberry is more likely to be eaten straight off the plant than make it into your front or back door. They taste so good!

## Additional Benefits

## Connection to nature

So many people say their lives are harried, hurried, and stressed. Under the barrage of texts, emails, phone calls, appointments, classes, meetings, and updating your online status, there is no time to relax and enjoy life. Gardening gives you that chance.

Not only do you benefit by having healthy edibles, just outside your door, but you also get to feel like a part of something greater. When you consider what a miracle it is that one tiny seed can grow an entire head of lettuce, a bush loaded with tomatoes, or a crawling vine that pumps out beans like some kind of unstoppable machine, you cannot help but be amazed and awed.

Nature is amazing. It has powers we can only dream of. Yet we, too, are a part of the natural world. When we cut a finger, we heal without doing anything. We sprout from two microscopic "seeds" and grow into something that can move, speak, create, make music, play games, build structures, and change the world.

Gardening helps connect us to that natural, miraculous part of ourselves. It reminds us of how amazing we can be, and how we fit into a larger puzzle, just as plants, animals, microorganisms, water, and sunlight fit together into a larger ecosystem.

## Respect for what you grow

When you finally get your first lettuce, after having to figure out what has killed all the seedlings you've been planting, and you taste that delicate, sweet crunch, you savor it more than you ever could a head you grabbed from a store shelf before rushing home to make dinner. When you have finally built your soil to where it holds moisture and provides nutrients for your plants, set up watering systems to be as efficient as possible, then eat your first string beans, you appreciate them more than any you could ever buy.

Your garden becomes payment for your energy, labor, research, devotion, and patience. When you work to get your food, you appreciate it more, because you understand how much goes into producing it, and what a miracle it is you got food at all.

## Seasonal eating

Much of the produce in stores has been shipped from other parts of the country, and even from other parts of the world, so that we can have, for example, some tomatoes in the winter, even though tomatoes are a warm-weather, summer crop.

Produce loses more nutrients the longer it has been since it was picked. By picking and eating your own food, you eat what's in season, and what's fresh. That translates to tastier, healthier food.

# A plethora of choices

In a store, you have maybe four or five varieties of lettuce, one type of carrot, three choices of onion, one kind of green bean. But there are thousands of varieties of fruits and vegetables that have been developed and preserved all over the world. You get to tap into that when you grow your own food.

How about 56 types of lettuce--everything from tight, crisp heads, to antler-like leaves, to red-freckled green? Imagine your next tossed salad with the crunch of pink, salty Swiss chard stems, frilly, delicate, licorice-like fennel fronds, bursts of sweet, juicy tomatoes, and sharp, peppery, burnt-tire-like arugula. Wow! That's quite different from the salad you can get at most take-out places or even restaurants, where the standards are green iceberg lettuce, mushy tomatoes, and maybe some stiff carrot shreds.

Speaking of carrots, how much fun would it be to grow purple, yellow, and white carrots, instead of orange ones? Or green-striped, yellow peppers, or fingernail-sized tomatoes, some tangy, some mild, some candy sweet?

There are different colors, shapes, sizes, flavors, and aromas, even within one vegetable. Some of the greatest variety can be found in tomatoes, eggplants, and peppers. Tomatoes can be round or elongated, palm-sized or in clusters like grapes.

Eggplants can be purple, green, white, or have orange and yellow stripes. Peppers can be curved like a bird's beak, or scrunched up like an old man's face. They can be sweet as a melon or hot enough to make you want to die.

Ever seen a kale leaf bigger than your head, or a squash larger than a baseball bat? I have, in my garden, and you can, too, in yours.

## Get exercise and fresh air

You will be out in the fresh air when you garden, moving your body without realizing it, as you dig, weed, plant, harvest, haul, and water. There are days when I have nothing to harvest, nothing to water, and yet I still find myself drawn outside, just to be among the plants, enjoying them. Often I get sidetracked, spotting a praying mantis perfectly camouflaged, or a lizard doing pushups to look tough for another lizard. Or excited when I spot some new peppers, beans, tomatoes, or cucumbers that may grow into plump, juicy fruits.

Even the most practical-minded gardener, who starts out wanting nothing more than to produce food, will end up appreciating more than just the harvest. Nature has a way of seeping into your soul, nourishing and replenishing it, often without you even realizing it. Gardening is a productive way to connect with nature and get some exercise at the same time.

## Feel a sense of pride and accomplishment

I must admit it is a bit of a rush when someone stops to admire my garden as they are walking by. Sometimes it's mostly weeds and needs a lot of work, yet the swath of greenery with pops of color from flowers (often weeds!) catches their eye.

You can look at an armful of freshly-picked greens, or a basket full of tomatoes and green beans, and be proud of the fact that all of it happened thanks to your efforts. Gardening is not easy. Many people try it; few continue to do it, because there is so much that can go wrong, and patience and knowledge are required.

But so much can go right, and when it does, you are there to witness it. You get a sense of accomplishment, knowing all those nights going out to kill the slugs made those juicy strawberries, free from toxic chemicals, possible.

## Great to get kids involved

Gardening is a fantastic activity for children. They have an innate curiosity and powers of observation that are rewarded by spending time in the garden. They can watch bugs, dig for worms, and look for weeds.

Kids love to help spot a ripening tomato, or a camouflaged green bean hidden amongst green leaves. They do not balk at exercise if it involves unearthing potatoes or pulling up a stubborn daikon.

Many schools have implemented gardening programs because it not only provides a real-life classroom where they can learn about ecosystems, the water cycle, and biodiversity, but because it helps with nutrition. Kids are more likely to try new foods when they have had a hand in preparing them. And what kid could possibly resist tasting something as funny-sounding as a cassabanana, kohlrabi, or snake gourd?

Working in a garden teaches children the values of persistence, observation, and patience. They must use restraint, discipline, and detective skills. They can get a sense of order and accomplishment by taking charge of their own section of the garden. Allowing them to choose what they want to grow gives them a chance to make decisions for themselves, which is hard when you live in an adult-controlled world. And they also get to learn about the consequences of their choices and actions.

When a child chooses to plant sunflowers in a shady spot, or puts too many seeds close together, they can learn, when their plants don't fare so well, that choices have consequences, and they may be more careful in the future. All of these are lessons we need kids to learn, but gardening can provide an opportunity to teach them in a way that is more fun than hearing a lecture from an adult, or a warning from a teacher.

Children are sponges, eager to learn. Kids who have the chance to learn from nature when they are young have more respect for it and are more likely to carry those skills and knowledge into their adult lives.

When my siblings and I were growing up, we were constantly dragged to orchid shows, plant sales, and nurseries. Much of the time we whined about how long Mommy took to buy something, and how thirsty we were and wanted to go home. But as adults, all three of us are avid gardeners, with fruit trees, orchids, vegetable gardens, water lilies, and plants galore. Who says nothing rubbed off?

# CHAPTER 2

## How Does Nature Do It?

Nature has survived for millions of years without human intervention, yet modern societies think we are smarter than that. Mechanized farming is the predominant model used to produce our food today, yet this system is failing.

Individuals have taken a stand, and backyard gardening is on the rise. More people than ever before are learning how to grow their own food, using nature as a model.

If we study the way nature produces food, we need to look at areas where fertility is high, and human intervention low, to find out why. And then we can apply those principles to mimic the wisdom nature already has.

### Growth in a forest

Imagine yourself in a forest, woods, or jungle. Trees abound, but nobody comes in to prune, water, or spray them with chemicals. The floor is littered with leaves, decaying branches, and insect life. Nobody comes to blow the leaves, pluck the weeds, or kill the nasty bugs.

Yet life abounds. And it does so regardless of the seasons. There is as much life visible in the winter as in the spring, even though, in colder areas, some trees go dormant.

### Life in a desert

What about the opposite--a dry, barren desert? There is only a fraction of the rainfall every year that exists in a rainforest, yet there is still life everywhere. Plants take on different forms. They have adapted to drier conditions, with small and thick leaves that withstand temperature extremes, and deep taproots that bury to find limited moisture.

Yet even here, things thrive. The animals have found ways to adapt. Lizards bury themselves in the sand to escape the punishing heat. Spiders and beetles gather dew in the early morning light on their webs and bodies, and drink them to survive.

## The basic principles

Forests, savannahs, or deserts--all have several principles in common. They maintain the living ecosystem and keep it healthy, even with climate change and natural disasters.

## Everything is recycled

Unlike with commercial gardening, there are no crop-dusting planes flying overhead, spraying tons of toxic chemicals to kill insects, provide nutrients, and prevent disease. Whatever dies stays right there, and its nutrients break down in the soil, creating sustenance for the next generation of life.

## There is minimal input

Nobody comes in to tidy things up. Trees bend and shape to reach adequate sunlight, twist and thicken to withstand wind, and only the healthiest survive. Those plants and animals that cannot live in these conditions die and are replaced by others that can.

Whatever is, is. Nothing is designed to look a certain way, fit into a specific space, or have a certain color scheme.

There are no bags of vermiculite, water-holding polymer crystals, or sterilized potting soil added regularly. None of the plants gets a regular dousing of 10-10-10 fertilizer or a side dressing of Super Duper Miraculous Plant Food. Nutrients come from the variety of plants and animals that live and die there.

Microorganisms in the soil itself break dead stuff down into nutrients, then help the plants absorb them.

## Plants have adapted to local conditions

There are no cactus plants in the rainforest, and no banana trees in the desert. But there are palms in the desert, and plants in the jungle that never touch the ground.

Species in any ecosystem have evolved to thrive there. They have learned to deal with any natural weather conditions, including dust storms, drought, hurricane, and flood. They are adapted to the temperature fluctuations and the amount of available sunlight and rain.

## Water is used effectively

Every plant and animal that exists on this earth needs water in order to survive. But the amount of water in any area differs from any other. Even in Hawaii, where you think of balmy breezes and sandy shores, there is great variation in climate and weather.

Some parts of the islands are dry like desert, with minimal rainfall every year. Other parts are rainforest, with tiny frogs, slugs, and spiders that live nowhere else on earth.

Drive for 20 minutes, and you can start to see moss on the sidewalks. Mountain valleys get almost daily rain. Near the ocean, hurricanes and tropical storms, plus near-constant sun and wind create a completely different weather pattern.

Yet in the natural bounty of each of these areas, water is needed by the plants and animals that live there, and they have adapted to take advantage of whatever amount is present.

Coconuts, for example, are perfect containers of water. Inside, liquid is stored and used by the seed until it can find solid ground and take root. In the meantime, the fibrous, outer husk provides shade, protection from attack and the elements, and a flotation device. Coconuts can float on the ocean with the currents, and when they get deposited on some new island somewhere, they sprout and grow, providing a source of food, water, fiber, and wood.

In desert climates, water is held in thin, needle-like, or thick, succulent leaves, which resist loss through evaporation better than the larger, flat leaves of plants found in temperate or tropical climates. Tap roots burrow deeply, because moisture and relief from the sun are found there.

## There is great biodiversity

Traditional farming methods grow field after field of one single crop, aligned in rows spaced evenly apart. This is known as mono-culture or mono-cropping, to make mechanized growing and harvesting easier.

Crops can be planted, fertilized, and harvested with machines that drive between the rows. Because the plants are all the same kind, they can all be sprayed with the same cocktail of chemicals, all at the same time.

In nature, there is a great mix of species, sizes, colors, and textures, all thrown together in a disorganized mess. Plants start to grow at different times and mature at different rates. Some use more of one nutrient than others.

Yet together they all form one compatible ecosystem. Often, symbiotic relationships occur between two different species, so that both benefit from the other. A typical example is the spreading of seeds by birds.

Birds eat the fruit of many trees, but the seeds do not get broken down in their digestive system. The bird flies to another area, poops, and out comes the seed. Often the acid nature of the bird excrement, plus the moisture in it, helps the seed to germinate in its new home. Without the bird intermediary, there would be no spreading of the seeds, and no new plants. Without the plants, the birds would have no food. But nature, in its infinite wisdom, has figured all this out already, and the cycle of continuing fertility has been taken care of.

Successful gardening comes from studying nature and how it works. By applying the principles that already work, we can develop mini-ecosystems and harvest from the bounty created in them.

# CHAPTER 3

## Real-World Proof

If you think barren, dry areas of the world that are unable to support life are destined to stay that way, think again. In many impoverished parts of the world, people in agricultural areas struggle to produce enough food from denuded soil. Yet there are several programs that have been developed, modeled after natural ecosystems, which have yielded tremendous results. Here are a few of them.

## China

The Loess Plateau in central China used to be one of the poorest areas of the country. People struggled to grow food in dry, barren land, and their herds of goats grazed what little was left of the mountains.

When it rained, the water washed soil away, causing floods. Silt swept into the Yellow River, clogging up the waterway and destroying villages downstream. In some areas, there were floating "mattresses" of mud, thick layers that floated on the surface, yet could not be penetrated, much like a waterbed, if you're old enough to know what that is.

Wind blew the dust into dust storms, polluting air in cities and other countries miles away. This became not only a local problem, but a national, then an international one.

Scientists and engineers concluded that human activity had caused this. The villagers, after generations of subsistence farming, had stripped the area of all its life. Their goats continued to denude what little vegetation managed to sprout. Now they were struggling to survive, tormented by flood, famine, and mudslides.

A project was proposed. A critical area would be developed to mimic the natural ecosystem that once existed. But the villagers were not convinced that planting trees on the mountains, and trees without fruits, to boot, would be useful.

"What good is a tree? My grandkids cannot eat trees," argued one farmer.

Eventually the villagers were convinced that not only would they have control over the area, but that they would actually benefit from this development. Farmers were paid to stop farming in certain protected areas, and to keep their goats penned up, so they would stop eating everything on the hillside. With government support, the villagers pitched in to make changes.

The tops of the hills were planted with trees, which capture rainfall and spread and hold it in the soil. They also provide homes for wildlife, which help with pollination and pest control. The middle sections were terraces, with food crops. The bottoms were converted to dams, to collect water.

What was the result of all that work? Was it worth it?

Fifteen years later, the entire area has gone from barren, lifeless desert, to lush, green mountains and valleys. Greenhouses produce so much food, the villagers sell it, and their income has tripled.

The soil has become rich with organic matter. It holds moisture and nourishes whatever grows in it. When it rains, the soil and plants absorb the water. There are no more floods or dust storms. There is much less silt in the Yellow River.

The region experienced the worst drought in history, yet it still produced ample food and water. Even with the changing climate nowadays, the people have food stability and can still thrive despite the hardships.

In fact, the project was so successful, that the Chinese government is repeating it in different places in the country. The environment benefits, and the people benefit and are empowered.

## Saudi Arabia

Rain used to fall three times a year in Al Baydha. But rain had been getting more and more scarce. Many aquifers were running dry. Wells were deepened to reach water. When it rained, the water created flash floods, taking soil with it and causing death, destruction, and damage.

Villagers raise animals and sell firewood as their main sources of income. The land around them was so barren, they were forced to buy feed for their animals. They were getting close to a tipping point, when they could no longer afford to feed their animals, and they would lose their homes and livelihoods because there would be no way to survive where they were. But a project to stop and collect water has already made a world of difference.

Earth berms (walls) were erected to trap water that comes off the mountain when it rains. The rain seeps under the soil and forms a seasonal stream, which can be used to irrigate plants. Terraces were built, using the plentiful rocks in the area, to slow the flow of water, reduce erosion, and create areas to plant in.

After the first rain, enough water was collected to plant and irrigate 1000 trees for four years. The next rainfall did not come for another three years, until 2014. When it did, enough water was collected to plant another 1000 trees and will be used to irrigate them for the next six years.

The Al Baydha Project is only beginning, but it has already made a huge difference. Trees are bearing fruit, and the plans are to produce a food forest that will provide food for people and animals, plus timber, mulch, and shade.

The ultimate goal is to teach the villagers other skills, such as operating a dairy, using goats that are better adapted to survive in their area. They are also learning all the principles involved in the current project, so that they can become knowledgeable and self-sufficient and can continue to make changes and shape their own lives.

## Ethiopia

The people of Ethiopia have struggled for a long time with civil war and conflict. In addition, half of the country is mountains, most of which are barren and dry. Generations of subsistence farming have left the earth denuded and lifeless. Just like in China and Saudi Arabia, when it rains, floods carry the water and soil away and case death and destruction.

The villagers of Abraha Aspaha had the choice: flee as refugees to try to find better circumstances, or stay and try to improve their situation. Many had already left. Many had died due to famine in 1984.

With help from the government, the villagers who stayed began to restore the ecosystem. Just five years later, changes are drastic.

Children can go to school, instead of walking miles in search of water, or working in fields to eke out food crops. Food is plentiful, and life is stable. They can grow more varieties of food than they could before, and the fruit trees are thriving.

Even with the unpredictable climate changes occurring recently, the village can tolerate them and continue to improve and grow. All of this because of people's efforts to mimic nature and bring back the natural balance.

## Change is possible

Regardless of whether you believe global warming, deforestation, mechanized agriculture, or other things are the cause of climate change and its unpredictability, one thing is clear. Change can happen when humans decide to work with nature, instead of trying to conquer it.

Warmer temperatures, droughts, and water shortages are happening already. You can decide to either argue about the causes, or do something toward a solution.

The rest of this book will show you principles, methods, and ideas you can implement in your own area. Use them to work toward your own balanced ecosystem, one which can provide you with abundance and food stability.

# CHAPTER 4

## The Big Picture

We need to look at exactly what happens to water and plants in regards to moisture. Then we can understand what is important when we try to apply these principles to gardening.

### What happens to water?

The first thing we want to consider when planning a drought-resistant garden is what happens when there is moisture. Some water runs off, some evaporates, some drains away, and some sticks around.

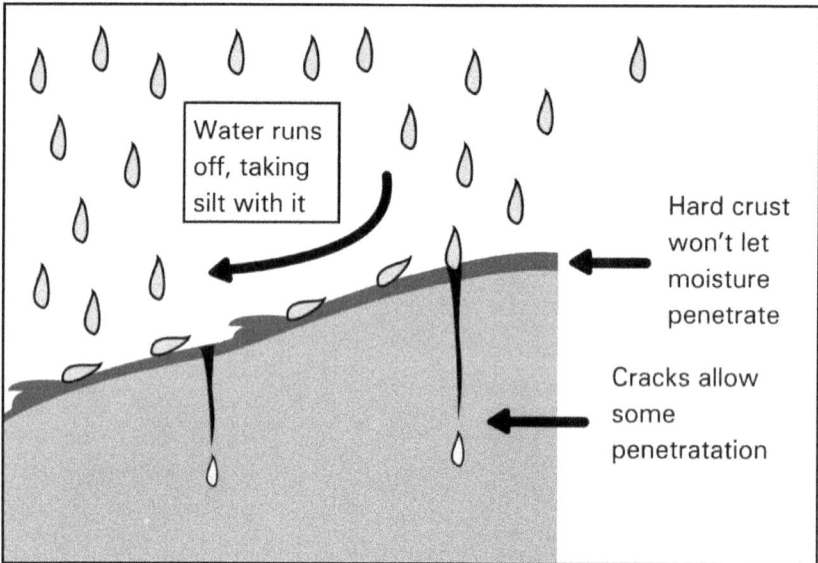

Water runs off, taking silt with it

Hard crust won't let moisture penetrate

Cracks allow some penetratation

In the case of denuded areas, where there is no vegetation to help contain the moisture, runoff can be severe, taking soil with it, causing mudslides and flooding, as we saw in the real-world examples in the last chapter. Also, the top layer of soil has often formed an impenetrable crust, from baking in the sun, so nothing can pierce the top layer and filter below. Cracks in the top crust allow some water to penetrate, but there is very little in the soil to sustain life.

In typical garden soil, when water falls, usually from rain or overhead watering, some of it is held in the soil, while most of it filters down and away. There is some runoff, but not as much as in barren areas, because plants absorb the moisture and slow down its movement.

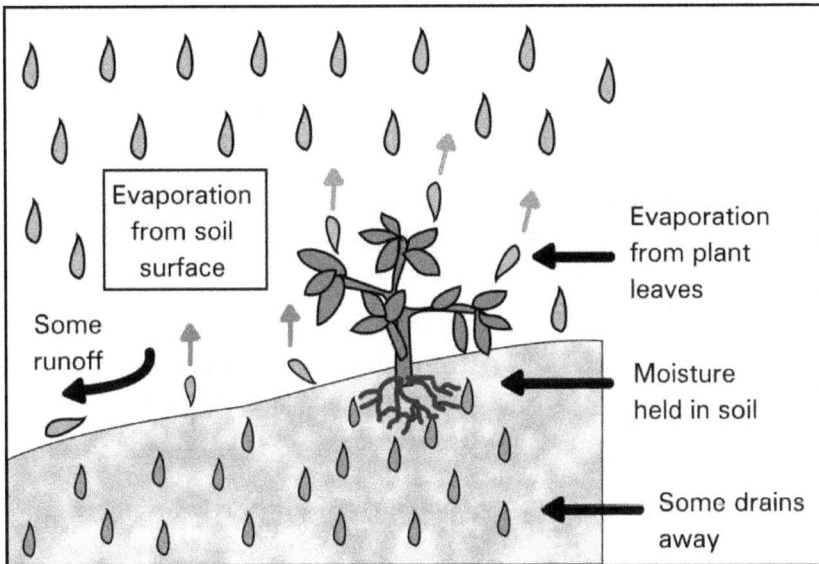

Some of the moisture evaporates from the top of the soil. And some is released from the leaves of the plants, which is called transpiration. Both of these types of evaporation can be speeded up or slowed down depending on how much wind and heat there is.

## What happens to plants?

Plant cells hold moisture in them like millions of tiny water balloons. When the plant is hydrated, the plant stands upright, and stems are firm.

When the plant is dehydrated, the water-balloon-like sacs are empty, causing the leaves to wilt, and the plant to droop. If this continues, it can cause permanent damage and ultimately, death.

## The solution for gardening in a drought

In order to make the best use of moisture during times of shortage, we need to be as efficient with our water use as possible. So we must attack the problem from different angles.

First, we will concentrate on holding more moisture in the soil itself. That means eliminating most of the wastage from runoff and drainage, by increasing organic matter.

Secondly, we need to reduce the rate or amount of evaporation, both from the plant itself, and from the soil surface. Mulching, shade cloths, and windbreaks do this. We'll also look at ways to reduce or redirect runoff.

Thirdly, we will look at watering and water conservation. How can you get more water to use for the garden? What are the most efficient ways of putting moisture where it is needed, at the root zone, around the plants?

Next, we look at water-wise garden types that will work in many situations--urban, rural, in the ground, or on the surface, using what you have available. And if you have enough land to make large changes, what are some methods of modifying the landscape to increase the water-holding ability of the surrounding soil?

Finally, we look at the plants to include in your garden. Which ones are the most tolerant of drought? How do you choose what and when to plant?

The more of these angles you attack, the more success you will have. Because every situation is different, this book cannot possibly give you the perfect recipe for success. But by using the individual ingredients, and adding a dash of your own ingenuity and experimentation, you have the best odds of coming up with a winning dish...I mean, garden!

## Permaculture and Natural Farming

Permaculture is a system of environmental design, developed by Bill Mollison and David Holmgren in 1974, that works with nature in a way that cares for the planet and other people. Permanent + agriculture = permaculture.

Natural Farming was developed by Masanobu Fukuoka, a philosopher and farmer in Japan. By observing nature, he was able to create a farm using no cultivating or weeding, very little labor, and no compost or fossil fuels. Yet the yields on his land were comparable to those of neighboring, traditional farms.

By designing systems of agriculture that mimic nature, both methods found ways to produce food easily and bountifully. By exaggerating what happens naturally, you can get phenomenal results in a very short period of time. An added benefit is that nature does most of the work, meaning you do less of it.

The idea is to take an area of land and make it produce food, hold water, and be full of life, in a way that is sustainable. In other words, it will become a closed system that doesn't need regular expenses of energy and raw materials.

If you look at any forest or woodland, American prairie, African savannah, or Australian bush in the natural world, this is what you get. Animals and plants live and die in a balanced system. The animals and plants have enough food and water.

It's when people come in that problems usually occur, because when humans need space to expand, that usually means they cut down the forest, pave over whatever is natural, build cities, pollute what little water remains, and continue expanding outward in a similar fashion.

Often, you find indigenous people who have survived for generations by working with the natural world. They have developed methods of growing food and working with their environment that keeps them fed, watered, and housed without destroying what already exists. Yet they often end up adapting "modern" methods, with disastrous results.

Using permaculture or natural farming principles in your yard or garden means you are mimicking the workings of nature, rather than fighting it. Instead of growing a lawn that needs constant mowing, fertilizing and watering, you grow ground cover that needs little or no care. And you use that area to grow food, to provide for you and your family.

Rather than planting a garden in the traditional method, which uses chemical fertilizers, sterile potting soil, and lots of watering, weeding, and work, you plant garden beds using lots of organic material that will break down and feed your plants as they do. In turn, what you grow can be put back into the soil, to provide more nutrition for what is to grow afterwards. You plant trees to provide you with fruits over decades, shade your living space, produce oxygen, and hold soil in place.

You also plant a variety of crops, so that even if your weather is suddenly hotter, colder, drier or wetter than normal, you will have something that survives, that will feed you and your family. You work with the land, taking advantage of natural sunshine and the way the water moves through your property, and use that to your advantage, rather than fighting it.

Insects, weeds, pests, and disease all have a way of balancing each other out. Your job is to observe and see how they do so, then assist in making things continue to happen naturally.

I'm not going to go into much detail about either of these methods. But if this seems like it makes sense to you, I encourage you to do more research and start experimenting. Check the "Learn More" section at the end of the book for some resources.

# CHAPTER 5

## The Dirt on Dirt

It's all about the soil. The soil is what holds the roots of a plant in place. Fungi in the soil encourage root system growth, which will keep the plant holding steady in the ground, preventing it from falling over during high winds.

Plants get moisture from the soil, to keep their cell walls plump, so that photosynthesis can occur. Plants also get nutrients from the soil, pulling up what they need to maintain healthy root, leaf, and fruit production.

Healthy garden soil will hold moisture in place, rather than allowing it to drain away immediately, so plants will have access to that moisture whether it's early in the morning, high noon, or late at night. Yet it won't keep the ground waterlogged, which can cause the plant to rot in place.

### Soil structure and composition

Soil is made up of ground-up particles of rock, plus organic matter, and a host of living organisms. Depending on where you live, your soil is likely to lean towards being more sandy or more clay in texture, although all soil has sand, clay, and silt (finely-ground particles) in it.

Sandy soils are made up of larger particles of ground-up rock. They allow water to drain easily, so they have little moisture-holding capability. This is great if you plan to grow desert-loving plants, but no so great for vegetable gardening, since most vegetables have higher water needs than succulents.

Clay soil, on the other hand, contains extremely finely-ground particles which hold moisture more easily, but that means it doesn't drain well and can actually cause problems due to too much moisture in the soil. Also, clay can be very difficult to work with, because it turns hard as concrete when dry, and sticky as paste when wet.

Adding organic matter is the answer for both these soil textures. Soil with a healthy mix of sand, clay, silt, and organic matter is called loam. All gardeners strive to produce a healthy loam, which vegetables thrive in.

Organic matter allows the soil to retain moisture, and it also produces humus, a glue-like material which causes the soil to clump. This is important, because it's not just water that plants need to grow. They also need air.

Air is easy to obtain around the stems and leaves, but the roots need to be able to move into air pockets in the soil, where they can get oxygen. That's why it's very important to never compact your soil or keep it waterlogged.

Compacting it squeezes out all the air pockets. Plant roots then have a difficult time penetrating the soil, and when they do, they do not find the oxygen they need. As a result, you get stunted, slow-growing plants that never live up to their full potential.

By ensuring there is enough moisture-holding capacity, plus enough air in the soil, we provide the most hospitable home for growth. But plants also need nutrients to grow. They get them from microorganisms, which we'll look at next.

## It's a living ecosystem

There is a balance between organic material, microorganisms, decaying plant matter, moisture, nutrients, and non-absorbent particles. An ideal garden soil, capable of supporting lush plant growth, has all these things.

But most people either have no soil, or very poor soil to begin with. So they go out and purchase potting mixes, many of which have been sterilized. This is supposed to kill any harmful diseases in the soil, allowing your seedlings to have a healthier life. Or so the marketing would have you believe.

One theory of good health, however, holds that in order for an organism to have better immunity, it needs to be exposed to multiple threats. Coddling a child or a plant by attempting to destroy all the bacteria around it is not only a futile endeavor, but it may actually be counterproductive.

On the other hand, exposing a child or plant to various diseases causes natural immunity to develop. Rather than making an organism weaker, exposure to diseases can cause that organism to become stronger, assuming it survives the attack.

## We are not humans

We are surrounded by bacteria, fungi, parasites, and other microorganisms. They live on our skin, inside our gut, and in the air. They are so numerous that Bonnie Bassler, Chair of the Department of Microbiology at Princeton University, says there are ten times more bacterial cells at any time on or in a human being. "You think of yourselves as human beings, but I think of you as 90 or 99% bacterial."[4]

Scientists know only a tiny bit about how bacteria work. But we do know they are more complicated than we can figure out, there are countless species of them, and we need them to survive. They keep us alive, forming an invisible protective shield around us. They make vitamins and digest our food. At the same time, some of them can seriously harm or even kill us.

By using antibacterial soaps to try to kill off only the harmful bacteria, we just create more problems. In the first place, we cannot target some kinds of bacteria and spare others, nor can we get rid of all the bacteria. In the second place, attempting to

---

[4]Bonnie Bassler, TEDEd, http://ed.ted.com/lessons/how-bacteria-talk-bonnie-bassler (accessed April 24, 2014).

do so allows the bacteria to mutate. Bacteria that change just enough to survive an attack against them then become resistant to those chemicals, and they reproduce. Future bacteria are now stronger than they were before and are even harder to kill.

Humans are complicated collections of living organisms that work in well-orchestrated detail that we have only begun to understand. The same can be said of plants, the soil, and the organisms that live there.

We know just a tiny bit about them and their interdependent relationships--barely enough to understand that they exist, but not enough to fathom how or why. But we do know the soil is a living ecosystem, and that when we manipulate it too much, we can actually destroy that delicate balance and cause harm.

Commercial farming methods involve tilling the soil with machinery, which creates a temporary burst of nutrient availability. This is because you are disrupting the complex system of underground life when you mix layers up, killing soil organisms in the process. All of that leads to a long-term reduction in productivity, the opposite of what we think we are doing when we dig up an area.

Life in the soil is complex. Organisms in soil include bacteria, protozoa, fungi, algae, nematodes, rotifers, springtails, mites, earthworms, slugs, snails, and many insect groups.

Some of these organisms are harmful to plants, but most of them play an essential role in the health of the soil, breaking down organic and inorganic material, and making nutrients available to plants.

In one teaspoon of healthy soil, there are over one billion bacteria, 900 feet of fungi, 50,000 protozoa, and several dozen nematodes.[5]  The soil microbes allow all the nutrition that plants need.

In return, the energy the plants produce through photosynthesis goes back into the soil, where the microbes use them to survive. It's a natural, mutually beneficial, relationship.

So if you start to build your soil using sterilized potting mix, you are working on a barren foundation.  Also, many of them contain additives such as peat moss, which are harvested from an area of the world to such a great extent, that the ecosystem there is in danger of collapsing.

## Be like the forest

Remember our discussion from earlier, about what happens in a forest ecosystem?  Anything that dies falls to the ground, decomposes, and is used as nutrients by the next generation of growing things.

We can build healthy garden soil by attempting to mimic those same conditions.  In other words, find yourself some organic material and get it to break down.

## Compost, aka "Black Gold"

Compost is basically soil made from broken-down organic matter.  It's a human way of controlling and sometimes speeding up the process that happens naturally.

You can make your own compost or buy it already made. But it is essential to help provide nutrients and to hold moisture in the soil.

This is important if you are growing most vegetables and fruits. Most herbs, on the other hand, can survive on less "cushy" soil, and adding compost is usually not beneficial or necessary.  In

---

[5]  Marylin McHugh, *Seeds of Permaculture--Tropical Permaculture*, https://www.youtube.com/watch?v=2cr10nOm0xU (accessed April 24, 2014).

fact, many herbs are plants that have adapted to harsh conditions and prefer poor soil that does not hold moisture. So do your research before adding compost to any soil where you plan to grow herbs or succulents, such as cacti. You may be doing more harm than good, in those cases.

## Composting in a nutshell

Basically, you mix together organic material, such as vegetable and fruit scraps, straw, egg shells, coffee grounds, shredded newspaper, unwaxed cardboard, wood shavings, old plant material, grass clippings, leaves, and manure from poultry, horses, rabbits, sheep, goats, or cows. The mixture needs to be moist but not sopping wet.

Ideally there is enough of it to create a pile at least 3 feet (0.9 meters) wide by 3 feet high by 3 feet deep, but even that is not a requirement. It is either mixed often, or allowed to sit there undisturbed, and eventually, nature will do its magic. All the stuff you started out with will have broken down into a pile of dark, moist, rich compost, full of earthworms, bugs, microorganisms, and nutrients. It can then be added to your garden or used as mulch on the soil surface (more about mulches later).

Some people worry about the ratio of carbon-rich material, such as leaves, to nitrogen-rich material, such as grass or manure. You want to shoot for a ratio of 30 parts carbon-rich material to 1 part of nitrogen-rich material. In other words, 2/3 of your pile should be brown things, and 1/3 should be green things.

But if you get that wrong, you will probably still end up with compost in the end. It might take a little longer, but it will happen. You can also throw in some finished compost, to add a dose of microorganisms, but even that is not necessary, since there are bacteria and fungi in and on all living things.

Mixing in more nitrogen-rich material causes the pile to heat up faster, resulting in faster decomposition. But some believe doing so also burns up nutrients and should be avoided.

Turning the pile with a shovel, pitchfork, specialized tool, or using a commercial "tumbler"-type of container helps the material to break down faster. But that also means more work for you.

Breaking the material into smaller pieces helps it break down faster. Adding stuff to the pile mixed together initially, instead of in layers, helps it to break down faster. Allowing your chickens to scratch in the pile helps to mix it up more.

You may choose to use human urine in the pile, which is a source of nitrogen. Some people collect their urine and mix it in. Others pee on the pile. Some find the whole thing too disgusting to even consider.

Whatever you choose to do, avoid adding cat or dog manure. These can contain harmful organisms, which can then make you or your family sick.

If you decide to add scrounged materials from outside your property, know that you can inadvertently ruin your compost or soil. Some people have horror stories to tell of "killer compost" that they traced to pesticides used on something they picked up elsewhere and added to their compost piles. Rather than supporting growth, the finished compost killed their gardens and poisoned the soil for years afterwards.

Avoid the temptation to pick up free manure from horse stables or discarded bags of leaves and grass clippings from other houses you may drive past. Unless you're sure the material, including the horses' feed, has not been sprayed, pass it by.

There is more information on killer compost, plus directions on how to test for it, if you think you might have picked up something harmful, in *Chapter 11, General Gardening Tips.*

## Option One

Place organic material in a pile somewhere, wetting it as you go. Leave it alone for a year or so. It will naturally break down into rich, usable compost.

## Option Two

Use any number of composting systems or methods to produce a finished product in as little as two weeks. If you live in an apartment with a small space, you can use a commercial tumbler, which is like a barrel that spins.

You add kitchen scraps, weeds, shredded newspaper, etc. and turn the barrel to mix the materials. Eventually you get finished compost.

There is also a countertop commercial option available that uses a closed container for your kitchen scraps. You sprinkle some microbial starter to help with the decomposition. Eventually you end up with usable compost.

## Option Three

Skip the work and go buy some already made.

# What's free and fabulous?

Wood chips or tree mulch are the shredded branches and trunks of trees and bushes that have been run through a powerful machine and broken down into smaller pieces. You can apply them on top of the soil as mulch.

Do not mix the chips into the soil, because they need nitrogen to break down. If you mix them into the soil, growth of your plants will be severely stunted. Leave the chips on top of the soil, where they prevent evaporative loss and help to soak up moisture, especially once they have started to break down. An added bonus is that as they break down, they provide nutrients to your plants.

To get chips, you can sign up online at ***chipdrop.in***. Or try and contact tree trimming services. You will likely find some who would be more than happy to dump a truck load of wood chips on your property. No need to pay them. You are doing them a favor, since they normally pay a fee to dump this material at a landfill or greenwaste facility.

The downside of having a pile of chips is that you get whatever is in the load at the time. The first time I got a load, it was full of thorns, because the trimmers had been cutting some roses and lauhala, a tropical plant with sawtooth-like edges on long leaves resembling palm fronds.

Also, there is likely to be mold in the pile. Therefore, you should avoid handling it or breathing the dust, particularly if you have asthma or other respiratory problems.

Beware that you could be introducing new pest species or diseases to your garden. Chinese rose beetles accompanied the rose debris in the last pile we got. The chickens and ducks loved eating the plump grubs, but we did have some damage from the adult insects who survived intact.

Keep in mind that the amount dumped is enormous. One pile is usually larger than your car. You need a place to put it and keep it for the year or so it will take to break down into usable compost.

Finally, know that the chips will wash away in heavy rain, or blow away in strong winds. So this option is best for people with large areas of land where the chips can be dumped and left alone, away from complaining neighbors' eyes, and out of the way. There it can miraculously go about its business of turning into tremendously fertile compost.

Despite the drawbacks, I find this to be one of the most beneficial ways to add organic material to the garden, with tremendous results. Plants seem to love the finished compost, and you can't beat the price, which is free! There are some gardeners who use little more than wood chips and rock dust, chicken manure, or other sources of nitrogen as fertilizer, and swear by the results. (Find out more in the next chapter).

## Wriggle while you work

Raising worms, or *vermiculture*, is all the rage these days. You feed the worms food scraps, shredded newspaper, and cardboard, and they produce rich, fertile "castings" (which is just a nicer word for "manure"), which can be added to the soil. They also produce moisture called "worm tea," which can be added as you would a liquid fertilizer or spray.

The downside to raising worms is that they need maintenance, just like pets do. You don't have to walk them, and they never make too much noise, but their beds need to be cleaned out periodically, and they need to be fed daily, or they will die.

If you think this might be something you're interested in, ask at a local garden center or nursery. They are likely to know someone who sells worms and can get you started.

It's a good idea to learn about vermiculture before you jump into it, however. So get yourself a good book, or find a forum with helpful discussions, to see if this will match your lifestyle. You can also find classes in your area, and these often include a live, working worm bin example, so you can see and smell the process for yourself.

## Your throne of fertility

That's right. Organic matter includes human feces and manure. In primitive societies, this waste matter is often used as "humanure" to fertilize crops.

However, there is potential for the spread of disease, so you need to proceed with caution. One way to take advantage of your own waste, however, is by using composting toilets.

Some you can build yourself. Others are commercial models. The basic principle is the same as backyard composting--the organic material breaks down over time.

Solids are often separated from liquids. Urine can be used in a backyard compost pile or diluted with water and sprayed on plants. Use 20 parts water to 1 part urine and apply to your foliage no more than once every few weeks.

Just like with other organic material, avoid using urine or manure from humans who take medications or are undergoing chemotherapy or other chemical treatments.

Flushing body waste using clean water is probably the greatest waste of water in a developed society. It is estimated that the average household flushes away one third of all the water they use, down the toilet. Even if you decide not to compost your human waste, consider ways to reduce the amount of clean water you flush away. (See Chapter 7 for more water conservation tips and tricks).

## You scratch my roots, I'll scratch yours

Mycorrhiza is a symbiotic, or mutually beneficial, relationship between a fungus and plant roots. The fungus helps the plant to absorb more nutrients and moisture from the soil, withstand drought better, and become healthier plants.

The fungus produces hyphae, root-like strands that infiltrate the soil around the plant's root zone, sticking to and wrapping around the plant's roots. This helps keep moisture and nutrients around the plant, where they are needed and used.

The plant helps the fungus by providing carbon that is used for growth and development. The fungi cannot produce sugars on their own, but the plants can, so they share these nutrients.

Mycorrhizal plants have been studied for 25 years by Texas A&M University, and gardeners are just beginning to learn about these naturally-occurring relationships. They show potential to help fix soil contaminated with petroleum products and heavy metals, so they may be increasingly useful in future oil spills, for example. Mychorrhizal fungi develop naturally where there is a lot of organic matter; you don't need to add anything specifically, if you'd rather not.

Or you can apply mycorrhizal products when sowing seeds, transplanting seedlings, or preparing beds for planting. Apply as directed and work it into the top 4 to 6 inches (10-15 cm) of the soil.

Avoid tilling your soil or using synthetic chemical fertilizers, which destroy the microorganisms. And don't bother using them on blueberries, azaleas, spinach, beets, turnips, radishes, or brassicas, such as cabbage, broccoli, kale, mustard, cauliflower, kohlrabi, and Brussels sprouts.

Those plants do not form a relationship with the fungi. They ignore each other. They are not on speaking terms. It's like two people who turn the other way when they see the other one heading towards them in the supermarket. What--me, antisocial?!!

## Work less and get better results

Tilling, or turning over the layers of soil by digging deeply and mixing the soil up, is discouraged. It breaks up the hyphae networks that help your plants withstand stress and drought. It also kills soil organisms and throws the natural balance off kilter.

Instead, break up the soil only at the surface, if you must. Stick to the top 4-6 inches (10-15 cm). But if your soil is hard and compacted, you can use a fork to get deeper. Rather than throwing the mixture onto the soil surface, merely rock the handle of your fork back and forth, to loosen the soil a bit.

You can also grow deep root vegetables, such as daikon, carrots, and burdock, which send roots deep into the soil, breaking it up. This will not destroy the soil ecosystem, yet still allow plant roots to easily penetrate.

Also, avoid compacting your soil. Never walk on growing areas. Use a large board or series of boards if you need to stand on a growing area, so that your weight is more widely distributed.

Maintain pathways through your garden and walk on them instead of your growing areas. Keep sections of your garden small enough that you can reach across to work and harvest, without needing to step into them. Doing so will keep your soil loose enough to support proper microbial growth and allow plant roots to grow more easily.

# CHAPTER 6

## Stop Spouting Off: How to Reduce Evaporation and Runoff

Once moisture is in the garden, whether it has arrived from rain, watering, or irrigation, keeping it where the plants can access it is important. Using compost and other organic material helps keep moisture in the soil, but we also need to reduce evaporation from above it.

One other consideration is reducing the amount of water that runs off slopes or impermeable areas. Rather than allowing it to flow away, you can reduce the runoff and/or channel it to growing areas.

### Transpiration

Plants constantly cycle through moisture. The tips of underground roots absorb water from the soil, and put it into circulation in the plant's vascular system. The moisture is wicked upwards into the stems and then the leaves, where they are important for photosynthesis, the creation of energy from sunlight.

Once water is in the leaves, it evaporates into the air, through a process called transpiration. To replace this lost water, more is pulled up from the roots, in a continuous cycle.

Some plants have adapted to low-water areas by modifying their leaves to reduce transpiration. Adapted leaves can be very small (as in the case of thyme), leathery, waxy, or covered in fine hairs. They can also be thick and needle-like. Examples can be found in cacti or plants suitable for a Mediterranean climate, such as the herbs rosemary and lavender.

The only ways to reduce water loss from transpiration are to either choose plants that are modified to survive in dry areas, or to increase humidity in the area. But increasing humidity is not easy to do when you are trying to reduce water usage, so we need to focus more on evaporation from the soil.

## Why water is lost

Most of the water is lost because of heat, dry air, or wind. Moisture on the surface of the soil acts like moisture in your clothes on laundry day. When you hang them on the line, your clothes will dry faster if the outside temperature is hot, it's a dry, rather than a humid, day, or if there is a breeze.

In the same way, soil moisture evaporates more quickly in warmer, drier, and windier areas. So to reduce evaporative loss, we can focus on providing a break from the sun, wind, and heat.

### Put a lid on it

Mulch is anything placed on the soil surface. It has multiple benefits. It traps moisture under it, preventing evaporation and making it available for your plants. This also makes the soil cooler, which helps some seeds to germinate. At the same time, mulch covers the ground so thoroughly that weeds are less likely to grow, and when they do, they are much easier to remove. Under the mulch, soil is easier to work, because earthworms are busy, processing the soil, and because the surface has not been baked into a hard crust by exposure to the sun. Mulching also helps to prevent diseases which can be caused by water splashing from the soil up to the undersides of the plant leaves.

You can use any number of organic materials, including grass clippings, wood chips, shredded leaves, or just more compost. Spread finely chopped material lightly around your plants, leaving space around each stem, to prevent rot.

In some circumstances, grass clippings and wood chips should be dried or broken down, although some people have used them successfully when fresh. The problem with fresh grass clippings is that they may harbor weed seeds, which can germinate and spread.

Large, whole leaves can compact when used as mulch, preventing moisture from penetrating the soil surface, so shred or chop all leaves before using them. You can do this by mowing them with your lawn mower, using a weed whacker (some people load them in a large wastebasket and put the weed whacker in there), or a leaf-shredding vacuum.

One gardener, Paul Gautschi, studied nature and decided to use wood chips as mulch in his garden. There is a film about his method, called *Back to Eden: Simple, Sustainable, Solutions*. The film focuses on the fact that he uses a very thick layer of wood and leaf chips on the top of his garden, but it fails to mention that he also adds manure from his chickens regularly. On his fruit orchard, he merely adds the tree chips as mulch.

He began using this system when there was drought in his area, and he couldn't water. He has found that he no longer needs to water, after years of adding chips continuously. His soil is exceptionally rich and moist and produces huge and bountiful harvests.

If you use wood chips as mulch, keep them on the surface. Do not mix them into the soil, or they will stunt growth. Some gardeners have had fantastic success piling on wood chips (mixed with leaves) at a depth of at least 4-6 inches (10-15 cm). In many cases, you may not need to water your garden, because the wood acts like a sponge, absorbing and holding moisture.

Chicken manure is high in nitrogen, making it a wonderful match for the chips. The two together will break down into a rich soil. You can try using another high-nitrogen source, such as grass clippings or human urine, to mix in with the wood chips as they decompose. But for most people, that's too much work.

Instead, you can leave the chips in a pile and allow them to decompose naturally. Once they have broken down, which takes about a year, you can mix them into the soil, where they will help to retain moisture and will continue to decompose.

The type of wood chips you have matters. It must be a mixture of green leaves as well as bark and branches. The green material contains sugars from photosynthesis and provides nutrients that will support life. Plain tree bark or wood shavings do not, and you will need to add other nutrients in order to get a balanced growing medium as it breaks down. But any tree trimmer will shred branches with leaves, providing the mix you need.

Also, be forewarned that if you use the wood chip mixture as mulch, you will probably not see good results the first year. As with other gardening methods (which will be covered in the next chapter), the material takes time to break down into usable nutrients for the soil. That's why it's recommended to start by adding compost into the soil, and using the tree chips as mulch. Eventually, they will break down and provide nutrition. In the meantime, your plants will get what they need from the compost.

Every situation is different, so you will have the fun task as a gardener of experimenting with different methods and ingredients in order to come up with a recipe that yields tasty results in your garden.

You can also do sheet mulching, using cardboard or layers of newspaper (do not use the glossy sections). Lay them on the ground, overlapping sections and leaving room for your plants. If necessary, place other mulch material on top of the sheets, to prevent them from blowing away.

Plastic sheeting, which will not break down, is often used in areas where you want to increase the temperature in a cold climate, so that heat-loving plants, such as melons, tomatoes, and peppers, will fare better. But it can easily cause overly hot temperatures, cooking your plants, so use it with care. Also, plastic does not break down in the garden into organic matter, so you will need to use your discretion on this.

Rocks can also be used as mulch material. One of the benefits to doing so is that they stay cool in the middle of any pile, so moisture in the air condenses on the rocks overnight and drips down into the soil.

Some farmers use this principle and stack rocks next to a tree, helping to water it. Also, a mass of rocks collects heat from the sun during the day and continues to radiate that heat at night. This helps trees that need warmth, such as citrus, to survive in areas that are normally too cold for them.

The biggest downsides to mulch are that they can blow around easily, smothering plants, and they can become a perfect habitat for slugs and snails to multiply. Areas that get a lot of moisture can be especially prone to this problem. If that happens, remove the mulch.

That's often a problem for us, because we have tropical storms that cause heavy rain for days or weeks at a time. Slugs and snails breed out of control, then decimate the garden. So the only thing we normally use for mulch is compost.

Before you add any mulch, water the garden or soil well, then apply mulch. Use mulch over any drip irrigation tubing. A layer of 4 or more inches (10 cm) is necessary to be effective. Add your mulch as early in the spring and fall as possible. Also, try to mulch before your annual weeds come up, or cut or mow weeds as low as possible to the ground, then add mulch. Do not pull up all the weeds with soil, since that breaks up the soil structure too much.

## Keeping your cool

Another way to prevent moisture loss is by providing shade. You can plant next to some sort of structure, such as a fence, the side of a house, a tree or bush. But if you do so, be sure the vegetables you choose can tolerate lower light levels. We'll discuss that when we look at what to plant (in Chapter 10).

Another option is to build a shade of some sort. This can be permanent, allowed to remain in the garden year round, or temporary, such as a cover put up during the hot summer months and removed the rest of the year. You might position your shade in the south, so it blocks some afternoon sun.

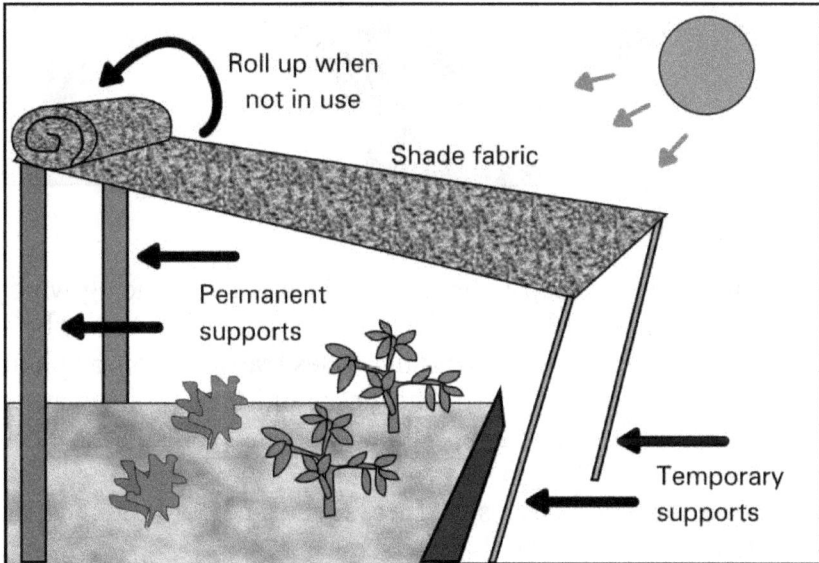

Shades can be made of shade cloth sold in garden centers, held up with wire, pipes, or other sturdy frame material, such as wood. They can be rolled back and tied in place when not needed.

Or you can make a support from large-mesh fencing material, onto which you direct vining and climbing plants to grow. The plants then act as the shade material. This works well if you have a small area that gets a lot of sunlight, and heat-and-sun-loving plants to train up the mesh.

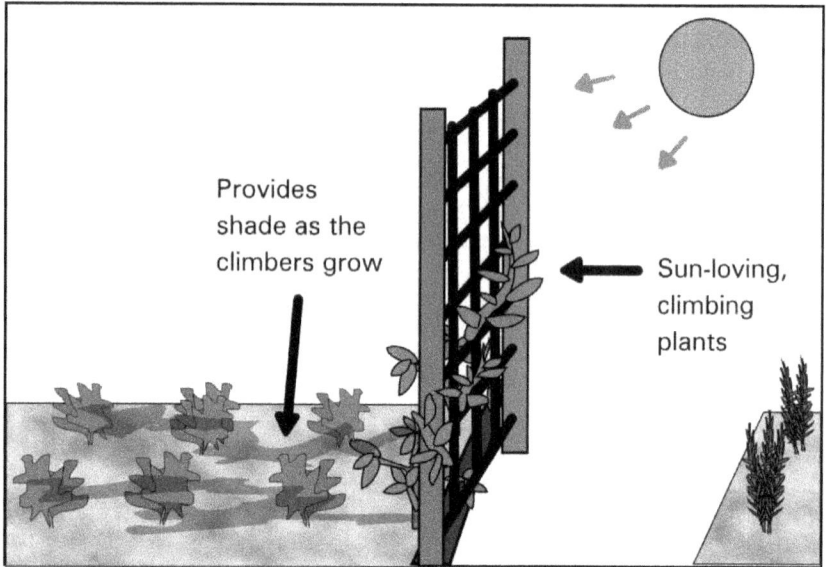

Provides shade as the climbers grow

Sun-loving, climbing plants

## Too much hot air

The third way to keep moisture in place is by reducing wind. You can attempt to block wind from your plants, but it may be a lost cause in some areas. Wind increases transpiration by plant leaves, evaporation from soil surfaces, and it also blows away mulch and can knock over or damage plants. Probably the most effective way to try to block wind is by planting near an already-established large structure, such as a boulder, fence, or wall, to decrease the wind's effects.

You may also choose to plant something to act as a natural windbreak, such as a row of trees, or even a single tree, bush, or large plants. Choose your plants depending on their moisture needs and what other benefits they could provide, such as food, wood, medicine, or attracting beneficial insects.

To be most effective, plant your windbreaks perpendicular to prevailing winds. They should be as tall and dense as possible.

Some examples of windbreak plants suitable for your garden are yarrow, comfrey, carrot, dill, and wormwood.

# Rolling, rolling, rolling:  How to reduce runoff

Another way to get and use water more efficiently is by decreasing the amount of runoff, the water that is lost by rolling off steep areas that are denuded of vegetation, or by passing over impermeable surfaces, such as asphalt and concrete.  By changing these surfaces so that water moves across them more slowly and down into the soil, you can retain moisture in the soil, where it seeps into surrounding areas, providing natural irrigation.

### The one time you want leaks

One thing that most gardeners can do is be aware of the type of surfacing you use for garden paths and stepping stones.  Instead of pouring a concrete slab, consider using permeable materials, such as gravel or wood chips, which allow water to filter down through them, into the soil below.

### Disconnected hard surfaces

Sometimes it is necessary to use hard surfaces, such as in a driveway, where a solid base is required.  In these cases, consider using disconnected pieces rather than one large, impermeable surface.  Instead of a solid area of cement, could you use large paving tiles instead?  Or cut the cement into sections, with small voids between them, to allow moisture to penetrate?

### Plan for runoff pathways

When all else fails, plan an "escape route" for water runoff. Rather than having all your precious rainwater flow from a cement slab into the street and eventually the sewer system, design so some of it can be channeled into growing areas.  It may be as simple as digging a small, narrow trench from an area of hardscape, to a planting area that is lower in the ground, so that gravity will naturally cause the water to flow downhill to it.

Or if you have a stone or brick border around a planting area just off a hardscape, you might be able to remove two or three bricks to create a similar channel for water to flow. A more elaborate system might include a channel at the lowest edge of hardscape, filled with drainage pipes that lead to your garden. Cover the pipes with gravel. Whenever it rains, that water will be redirected into your plants, rather than being washed away.

## Make it slow down

The most runoff occurs on sloped areas, especially where there is nothing to hold water in place. Where you have soil rather than hardscape or ground coverings, the best way to slow the water movement and reduce runoff is through plants.

Plants, including groundcovers, bushes, shrubs, and trees, use the moisture that comes their way. Their roots hold onto the soil so that it doesn't wash away in the rain or a storm.

Leaves and branches fall from the plants, providing nutrients for anything growing. This organic matter also provides shade from the sun, which can otherwise dry out bare soil and cause it to become impermeable.

By adding plants, you slow the flow of rain and allow it to seep into the ground, as well as spread the water around a larger area. Ideally, anything you plant would be drought-tolerant or drought-resistant once established, and if you can grow something that provides food, timber, or other useful materials, all the better.

Some of the plants in our yard I grow specifically to use as greens for flower arrangements, because I enjoy making them every now and then. Other plants have fragrant flowers, which are beautiful and add to our enjoyment and quality of life. But all of them hold moisture in the soil and prevent erosion.

Our property is on a gentle slope, and we used to have good coverage with grass, or whatever grass-like weeds that survived. But when we got chickens and ducks and allowed them to range freely, the chickens scratched most of those areas bare. I've watched the soil from the middle of the yard slowly move towards the back yard, and I'm in the process of transplanting some groundcover to areas of bare soil, so we don't lose it all. I can tell which plants the chooks and ducks leave alone, and some of them are both drought-tolerant and neglect-tolerant, which is important in areas of the yard where I don't do vegetable gardening. So I'll be relocating some of those plants to other areas, in order to reduce runoff.

In Chapter 9, Modifying Your Landscape, we'll look at specific ways to manage water by slowing runoff and spreading water flow throughout your property. In the meantime, consider what you have growing in your area, or keep these principles in mind if you are designing a new area, and see if there is something you can do to reduce transpiration and runoff, so that water stays where it can be used.

# CHAPTER 7

## The Fountain of Life: Water and How to Save It

Water is one of the primary needs of all living things. And vegetables use more water than most other plants in general do. So under water restrictions, you need to be careful of how much water your vegetable garden uses, and you must use that water in the most efficient way possible.

### Water conservation

Conserving water needs to be an everyday thing, not something we are forced to do only after shortages are imminent. If we wait until there is also scarcity, it becomes too late. Conserving water in the short term makes for long-term sustainability and abundance.

### Stop leaks

Look for dripping faucets, toilets that run, and holes in your irrigation tubing. Fix them.

### Turn off the tap

You don't need to run water when washing vegetables, brushing your teeth, or drinking. Fill up a glass and turn the tap off. Turn the faucet on to rinse your toothbrush and mouth, and turn it off while brushing. Fill up a pan or bowl and wash vegetables in it, then use that water to water your garden or flush your toilet.

When showering, turn on the water to get wet. Turn the water off to lather up, then back on to rinse.

You can buy shower heads with simple switches built into them. They are usually called "water-restriction" or "low-flow" shower heads, and they allow you to push a button or flip a lever, and the water shuts off at the showerhead. You wash your body, then flip the lever again, and the water turns back on. This eliminates your need for readjusting the water flow and temperature.

## Use water-wise shower faucets

There is a disturbing but very common shower faucet design that has one handle. It will only get hotter if you turn the water on higher. In other words, you cannot control the flow and the temperature of your water separately. It's very wasteful. Avoid installing this type of shower faucet, and consider replacing it if you have one in your bathroom.

There are designs that have two handles, or some with one handle, but with two controls, one for water temperature, and one for flow. Either of these two designs is more sensible and will save water, reducing your monthly bill at the same time.

## Re-use your water

Flushing a toilet is probably the greatest water waster. About one third of your home's water use goes to flushing. Rather than throwing away clean, drinkable water, reuse laundry water or sink washing water to flush with instead.

You can re-use any water to flush your toilet. Don't flush with the handle. Simply dump a quantity of water from a bucket or container held up high, into the bowl, so that the force of pouring the water causes your toilet to flush. Aim for the drain.

Even with mandatory, low-capacity toilets of 1.3 gallons (4.9 liters), that is more than one gallon per flush of clean water just going to waste. If you flush only four times a day, that's over 5 gallons (19 liters) of water gone. More than enough to water several containers of vegetables. And most people flush many more than four times a day.

Put a pan under your hands, or fruits and vegetables, when you wash them, to collect the water. Take a bucket with you into the shower. Any time you turn on a faucet and wait for the water to heat up, collect that water. It can be used to water your garden or flush your toilet, and it would normally just be lost.

Place a container under any air conditioner outlets outside your home. The dripping water can either be collected, or drip directly into plants underneath.

Never throw out any water if there is another use for it. If there is soap or detergent in it, it can still be used to flush the toilet. It might also be used in a graywater system, especially if you use natural cleaners.

## Your dirty water

Graywater is water that has been used in your home, including washing machine, shower, and sinks--anything except your toilet. The water, instead of being lost down your drains, is diverted outside the house, where it can be used for watering your plants.

Graywater can harbor dangerous bacteria, mostly from fecal matter in laundry machine water, especially if you have babies, children, or animals. But it also causes bacteria to grow, so it should be used that day and not saved for later, and not used on food crops.

You can have professional systems installed, or just divert your washing machine hose outside. One way to use it safely in the garden is to channel the water into an underground pipe between your garden beds. The water can flow out of the pipe, seeping into the soil, and your plants' roots can reach down into the soil to access the moisture.

Use natural cleaners if you plan to use graywater. To be safe, do not use graywater on edible crops, or parts of them that you will eat. In other words, don't water your vegetables with graywater. But you can water non-edible flowers and trees with it, or put it below ground, as mentioned above.

What about the soap--won't it kill the plants? In such dilute amounts, it does little harm. In fact, many people have found that it actually acts as a low-level pesticide, killing harmful insect pests. But definitely use natural cleaners, because you want them to break down in the soil, rather than killing microorganisms and causing long-term damage.

## Rain is nature's gold: How to collect it

In many places, there are rainy seasons or storms. You can collect that rainwater and have enough to water your entire garden for weeks to months afterwards.

Rainwater can be collected in large barrels made specifically for that purpose, or you can fashion a system yourself. Some people get barrels from food manufacturers and add spigots to the bottom so that a garden hose or drip irrigation system can be connected.

Keep in mind that any water collection that is used in this way needs to be gravity fed. So your water collection container needs to be higher than the area you're watering, in order for there to be enough water pressure to push the water through the hoses.

You can accomplish this by situating your water collection barrels uphill from your garden area. Or simply place the containers on bricks or sturdy stands to lift them off the ground.

Keep in mind that water is heavy. One gallon of water weighs just over 8 pounds (3.6 kg). One liter of water weighs one kilogram. Anything you use to support a container of water must be very strong.

If you cannot situate your water higher than your garden, you will need to use a pump to get the water where it needs to go.

Rather than connecting a hose to the barrel, you can simply dip a watering can or an old saucepan with a handle into the water to use for watering. Or if your barrel has a spigot, place your watering can under that, and use it like any other spigot as needed.

Rainwater can be diverted from a gutter system. There are diverters that can be installed to channel water into a barrel.

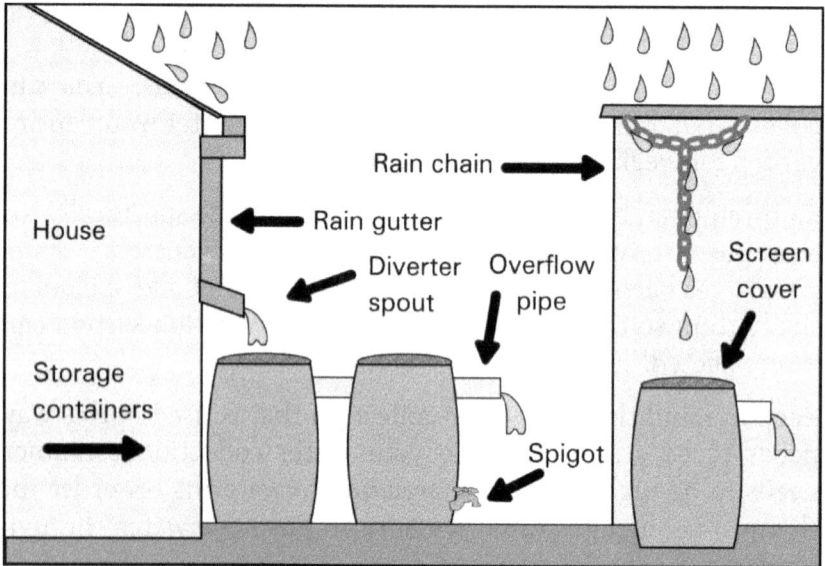

Or you can go as low-tech as a row of buckets under the edge of a roof, where water drips off. If you want to channel that water to a specific area, you can hang a length of chain from the edge of the roof. Water will flow off the chain into a container below it.

Barrels should have a screen covering so mosquitoes cannot breed in the water. It also helps keep debris out. Barrels also need a clamped-on or tight cover so children and animals cannot fall in and drown.

Be sure to add an overflow mechanism of some sort, which can be as simple as a hole drilled in the side. You can use tubing to connect several barrels together by attaching tubing to the overflow hole of one and putting the other end into the inflow of the next. One heavy downpour can produce a surprisingly large amount of rainwater.

## Low-tech high tech:  Fog collectors

Also known as fog fences, traps, catchers, or nets, these are basically a piece of fine mesh suspended on a frame. The mesh traps moisture in the air, and the drops gather together to form larger drops, which drip down into a gutter-like collection system at the bottom. Add filters to remove debris, and you have water to use for your plants.

Fog catchers are being used in the Atacama Desert in northern Chile, the driest desert in the world. It rains there only every four years. But the catchers are producing more water than the local people could ever imagine, and they are using it to reforest the area.

This technology is cheap and easy to use and maintain. It has been used in mountainous regions in South America and desert areas of the Middle East.

It works best in coastal, mountainous, and arid regions with lots of fog or mist. Limitations are mostly the size of the collection tanks and the length of the fog season. The system does double duty during the rainy season, collecting rainwater.

There are very few options to purchase fog collectors commercially, but you can probably make them yourself. Panels can be single or grouped together in rows.

String some nylon mesh between two vertical poles, so that the netting is taught. You may need to anchor the bases in cement, or tie guy-lines to provide more support. Each panel can be up to 516 square feet (48 square meters).

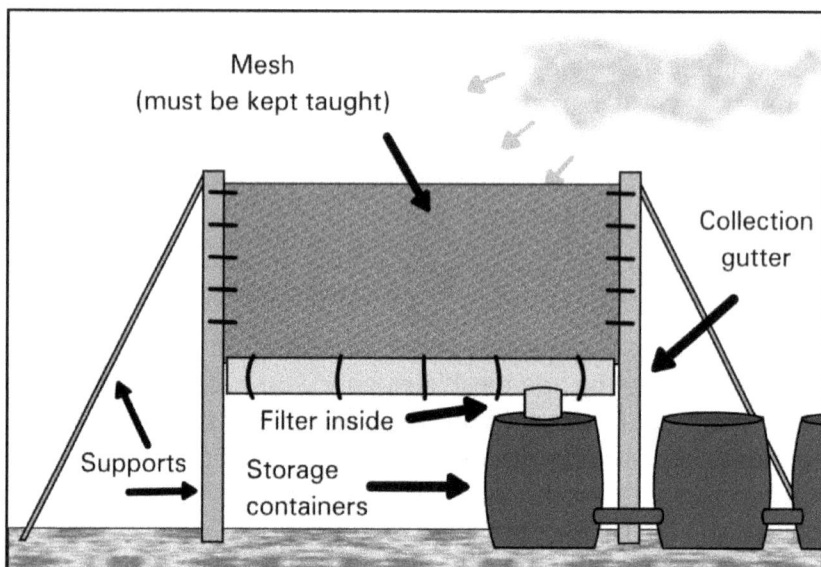

Attach a gutter, such as vinyl rain gutter, with one or two end caps, along the bottom. Add a downspout that empties into a collection container which is covered, to prevent mosquito infestation and evaporation. Add some window screen material or something similar inside, to filter sediment, insects, and other particles. Situate the panels perpendicular to oncoming winds.

The system is easy to use and maintain. Maintenance involves checking the panels for replacement when they have become worn, and scrubbing off any algae that grows (usually after one or two years) with a soft brush. You may also need to scrub out the gutter or tank occasionally with a chlorine solution.

You must keep tension in the fabric. Loose nets lead to a loss of efficiency and can break easily. Any tears in the mesh need to be repaired immediately.

I'm not sure if a special fabric needs to be used, but I'm guessing anything with a fine mesh, such as shade fabric or tent material, will work. There are not many people who have made systems like these at home, since the technology is relatively new and in the experimental stage. You'll have to be a pioneer and see what you can jerry-rig to work, if you want to make it yourself. See how it does in your area. If it works well, you can try setting up more.

Check the end of the book, where I list resources. There are some youtube videos with shots of systems in use. You can get some ideas for how to build your own, and see close-up footage of what the fabric being used looks like. It has triangular openings.

## Watering your plants

## Put it where it counts

To make the most efficient use of what water you have, you need to be sure that the water goes where it is the most effective. Since the roots are where moisture gets absorbed, that is where you should put the water.

The least efficient watering method is overhead, because most of the water ends up on leaves, stems, fruits, mulch, paths, and soil, and very little makes it down to the root zone. Most of that water evaporates, going to waste.

More importantly, the actively-growing root hairs at the tips of roots are where plants absorb water. So if your plant stops growing, it won't continue to absorb water, even if you give it more.

### Drip irrigation

Installing a drip irrigation (also known as trickle irrigation) system takes work and planning, but once it is in, water goes only to where you want it. You start by connecting a series of filters to your outdoor spigot. You can use a timer so there is minimal work on your part once the system has been set up and adjusted.

However, for maximum water efficiency, I recommend against using a timer. That way, you can turn your system on and off depending on how much rain, wind, and heat you've had lately. A timer just keeps pumping out water, no matter what.

You normally need to install a backflow device, to prevent water from your tubing flowing backwards into your water supply. Then a filter and water pressure regulator are connected, which transforms your high-pressure water source to a lower pressure, which is more efficient for the irrigation system.

An adapter connects to larger diameter tubes, which are set as a framework, and smaller, flexible tubes come off them. The smaller tubing can be soaker hose, which has tiny holes, that drip water out, spaced along the length of the tubing, or it can be solid and attached to a sprinkler or drip head. This can be spiked into the ground right next to a larger plant, such as a tomato plant.

The drawbacks to setting up a system are that you need to do some maintenance, such as repairing leaks, or replacing broken heads. You also need to be careful if you dig in your garden, so that you do not break any of the hoses. I mistakenly used a pick once to chop right through the large supply line when I was removing a fallen papaya tree.

Another drawback is that once you poke a hole in the tubing, you cannot remove it. So if you have set up a line in a certain spot, for example, you will always have to plant again in that certain spot. And your plants will need to go where the holes are in the soaker hose, which are spaced every 12 inches (30.5 cm) in our system. If a hole is not where you want to put a plant, too bad.

You can plug up holes you've made, but you cannot move things. That also means once your system is in place and you turn it on, it will water the entire area, regardless of whether you have anything planted there or not. Sometimes I have only parts of the garden planted, yet turning on the system waters the whole garden, wasting water.

There is also the overwhelm factor to consider, as well as initial set-up costs. It can seem quite complicated to set a system up, and you do need a fair amount of equipment.

But a drip irrigation system makes watering easy and efficient. Water goes directly to the base of the plants. If you do not have a timer, you turn your system on and shut it off later. Typically, systems need to run for only about 10-15 minutes.

## Ollas

Ollas (say "oh-yah") are the Spanish word for large vase-like vessels made of terra cotta. They have been used in central and South America as a non-automated drip irrigation system of sorts. Similar systems are used in Africa with dried gourds instead of terra cotta vessels, but the principle is the same.

The olla is placed into a hole in the ground so that the lip is flush with the top of the soil, then filled with water. Cover the hole in the top to prevent soil from falling in, mosquitoes breeding, and evaporation.

Because the clay is porous, moisture passes through the walls into the soil. When the surrounding soil is moist, water stops moving. As the soil dries out, water again seeps out.

One of the benefits of using an olla system is that the plants' roots go deeper into the soil to find moisture, eventually wrapping around the olla. This deep root structure helps to create plants that are more resistant to drought. Any deep-watering method will help to do this.

One of the drawbacks is that there is potential to break ollas when using farming tools.  Another is that they may break if you keep them in the ground over winter.

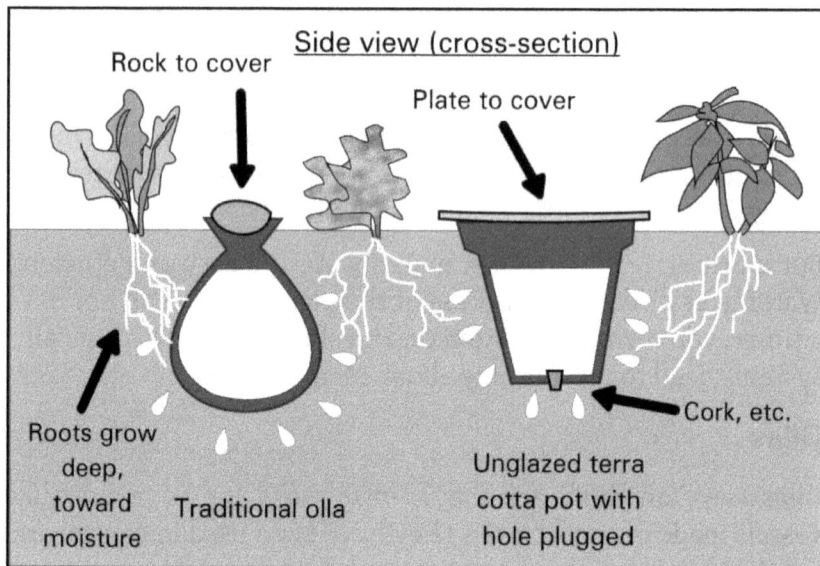

Side view (cross-section)

Rock to cover

Plate to cover

Cork, etc.

Roots grow deep, toward moisture

Traditional olla

Unglazed terra cotta pot with hole plugged

It is a good idea to keep them filled more than half full, rather than letting them get too low.  The salts and minerals in water that settle on the surface when water evaporates can clog the pot, making it less effective or useless.

You can use the olla principles in your garden by using traditional ollas, making them yourself, or substituting unglazed terra cotta pots or plastic milk jugs or beverage bottles.  You will need to poke a few tiny holes in the plastic bottles with a pin, since they are not already porous.

How far their reach can extend is uncertain, since there are so many different shapes and soil types.  As a general guideline, situate your plants so their centers are about half the diameter of the olla away from it.  So if you have an 8-inch (20 cm) olla, place plants with their centers within 4 inches (10 cm) away from the olla.

Ollas have been used for centuries in many places all over the world, including deserts. They place water exactly where it is needed and save water considerably.

## Terra cotta pots

You will need to plug the hole in the bottom of the pot with a cork, masking tape, or silicone caulking. Dig a hole into the soil to accommodate the pot, so the rim is flush with, or just above, the soil surface.

Fill the pot with water and cover it with a plate, to prevent evaporation and mosquito breeding. Check it often and refill it when the water level gets low.

You may need to occasionally scrub the pores of your pot with a stiff brush to remove any dirt or debris clogging the pores. And check your pots for cracks, which can cause water to leak out. Replace those pots.

## Beverage bottles and milk jugs

Use a clean bottle or jug with a cap. Poke several tiny holes with a pin or needle along the bottom and sides of the container. Dig a hole so the bottle cap will be flush with the top of the soil surface.

Put the bottle in the hole, fill it with water, and replace the cap. Water will seep out through the holes you made, mimicking the terra cotta ollas. You may need to do some experimenting with the size, number, and placement of holes you make, so that water doesn't just flood out and drain away too quickly.

Some people do not want to use plastic containers, because of the possibility that the plastic can leach chemicals into the water or soil. You will have to do your research and decide for yourself. Also, plastics tend to break down quickly in sunlight and may need to be replaced often.

But this method may be a good way to use what might otherwise get discarded or end up in a landfill. Also, there are methods you can try to link together two or more ollas using drip irrigation tubing. You can also connect the entire system to your rainwater catchment or other water supply. Or you may just decide to manually check each olla instead.

## Long pipes

A simple, low-tech way to get water to the root zone is to place a long pipe in the soil next to your plant. This works best with shrubs and trees. It can be a PVC pipe with holes cut into the sides, positioned to face the plant.

To water, you put your hose or spout of the watering can into the top of the pipe, which is above ground, and the water travels to the root zone, where the plant can use it.

Another take on this is to use a watering wand with the sprinkler head removed. Stick it into the ground next to your plants, and let the water run into the root zone. Pull the wand out and repeat with the next plant.

## Sub-irrigation

Sub-irrigation provides a chamber of water underneath the growing medium and plant(s). The plant's roots go deep, to get moisture, and the chamber is kept filled so that the plant has an unlimited supply.

Plants benefit by having as much water as they want or need. Water usage is reduced considerably, since almost none of it ends up elsewhere or evaporates.

In the next chapter, we will look at several sub-irrigation systems when we discuss water-saving garden types. But keep the principle in mind as you garden, and see if there are ways to use it in your situation.

## Water deeply

When you water less often and for longer periods of time, moisture goes deeper into the soil, causing the plant's roots to move deeper also. This creates a more robust, healthy plant that can withstand periods of drought.

On the other hand, if you water often and shallowly, your plants will do the opposite. Roots will remain near the surface, and any excess heat or drought is more likely to cause damage.

## When to water for the most benefit

If you water during the heat of the day, much of it will be lost to evaporation. Watering in the morning or late afternoon ensures that more of the water will stay where it is needed.

There is conflicting information about when to water. Some sources say not to water just before night, because then your plants just have wet feet and are more prone to fungal diseases. Some sources say water in the evening, because your plants do most of their repair and growing during the night.

Watering at night in arid places may be advisable, because it may give the water a fighting chance to soak in. And watering during the hottest parts of the day can be harmful to plants, because water drops can act to magnify the sun's rays, singeing leaves.

Obviously, you will need to see what works with your schedule and in your area. You might decide to water one section in the morning, and a different section in the afternoon, as an experiment, and see what happens.

Of course, this advice only applies if you use something like hand watering or drip irrigation, and not one of the constant water supply systems, such as sub-irrigation and ollas. Those have water available all the time, and the plants can do whatever they want. You're not the boss of them!

## How much to water?

It's all good and fine to say to water your plants deeply, but how much is that supposed to mean? Two minutes? Twenty five? Two hours?!

A typical garden needs 1 inch (2.5 cm) of water per week. But that is difficult to measure, and nearly impossible if you are using drip watering or sub-irrigation techniques.

You can place a pan under your drip system and stop after you've reached one inch. But probably the easiest way is to water until the top 6-8 inches (15-20 cm) of soil is wet. Time yourself to see how long your irrigation took.

The next day, stick your finger or a stick into the soil. If it is moist or soil sticks to it, it does not need to be irrigated. Or squeeze some soil into a ball. If it sticks together, it does not need to be watered. If it falls apart easily or barely holds together, it needs watering.

Irrigate when the top 2-4 inches (5-10 cm) is dry to the touch. Water again several times a week, if necessary, to the 6 to 8-inch (15 to 20-cm) depth.

The amount of water your garden needs will depend on many things, including the type of plants, temperature, how old the plants are, their state of health, how deep their roots are, how windy it is, and what time of day it is.

### Leaf wilting: It's not what you think

Some people think if your leaves are wilting, that is a perfect sign that your plants need water. This is not true. Plant leaves may wilt because they cannot absorb water fast enough, which can be a problem on very hot days. But too much water in the soil can also cause plant leaves to wilt. So how will you know if you need to water or not?

The best thing to do is to feel the soil in the root zone of the plant, the top 6-8 inches (15-20 cm) of soil. If there is obvious moisture, there is no need to water. If the soil is dry and your leaves are wilting, you need to water immediately.

Some leaf wilting will not hurt your plants. However, if continued, at some point, it will cause permanent damage or death to the plant. In fact, in some gardens that are heavily mulched, plant leaves wilt when temperatures rise but recover when it cools off.

However, if you see your plant leaves wilting in the morning or evening, they most likely need to be watered. Check moisture levels in the soil, and if it's dry, water.

## Container gardening

Plants in containers will need to be watered more often than plants in the ground. And plants in porous (such as unglazed ceramic or terra cotta) or smaller containers dry out more quickly than non-porous (such as plastic or glazed ceramic) or larger containers do.

Container plants may need to be watered daily in hot weather. When temperatures reach into the 100s, they may need twice a day watering. For most people, this is too difficult to do, so options such as sub-irrigation and olla systems are ideal.

## Germination and transplanting

Seeds need constant or near-constant moisture to germinate. Seedlings and transplants need frequent watering, especially after transplanting into a new area, to overcome the stress of moving, and to help establish new root growth.

Any transplants, even larger ones, including shrubs and trees, and anything considered "drought-resistant," will need watering until they get established. For most garden vegetables, two weeks is adequate. For trees, two years may be necessary.

## Factors needing more water

Higher temperatures, more sunlight, lower relative humidity, and more wind are the four factors, in order, that cause a plant to use more water. However, these four factors are often largely out of gardeners' control, as they vary with the seasons and the whims of nature.

Yet any measures you can take to change these factors, even if they only affect a tiny microclimate around your plants, can help to reduce water needs. Therefore, be sure to consider using shade cloths and windbreaks, as discussed previously, to see if they can help in your situation.

# Seed starting ideas

Here are some ways to start seeds. Basically, you want to allow constant, or at least, high levels of nearly constant moisture until the seeds have germinated.

## Simple and effective

This tried-and-true method works especially well for seeds that are hard to germinate. Place seeds onto a damp, but not soaking, paper towel. Lay another moist towel on top, creating a sandwich around the seeds. Place the sandwich in a zip-top plastic bag and seal it.

Keep the bag on a counter near a light but not sunny window. Check it after a few days, to see if the seeds have germinated. If so, carefully tear the towels into pieces that contain one seed each.

Transfer them into pots until they are large enough to transplant into the ground or larger containers. The towels will decompose in the soil eventually.

You will have better success if you wait until the seeds' roots have extended out a little, so they are stronger. But don't wait too long. The roots grow into the paper towel and are tiny and easy to damage when you tear the paper towel.

## If you eat out a lot

You can make a self-watering, seed-starting tray from some throwaways. Prepare your seed and paper towel sandwich as above. Place them in the bottom of a plastic tray with a fitted cover. Use a container from a takeout bento lunch or something similar. A clear cover is ideal.

Hold a small plastic drink bottle on top of the cover, and trace around the base with a pen. Cut an opening large enough to fit the bottle through the cover.

Poke a small hole in the bottom of the bottle with a pin or needle. Fill the bottle with water and replace the cap.

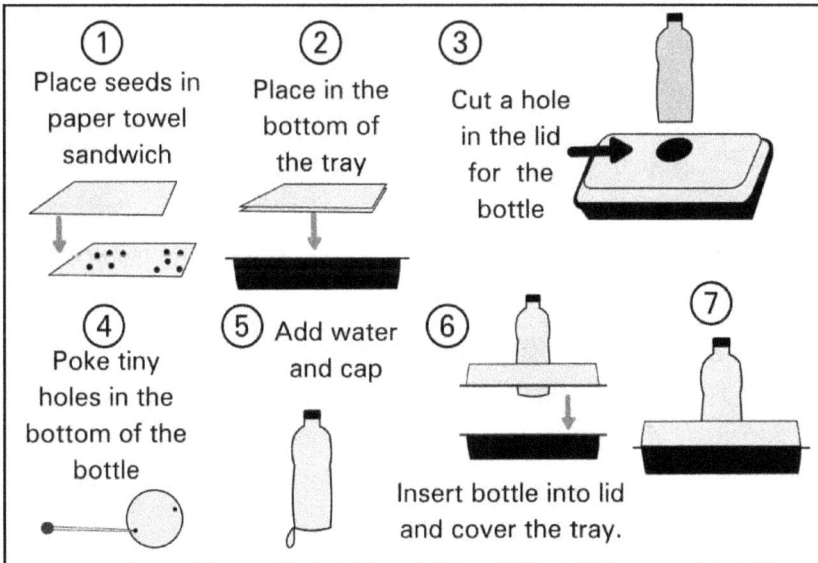

① Place seeds in paper towel sandwich

② Place in the bottom of the tray

③ Cut a hole in the lid for the bottle

④ Poke tiny holes in the bottom of the bottle

⑤ Add water and cap

⑥ ⑦ Insert bottle into lid and cover the tray.

Place the bottle through the hole in the lid, onto the paper towels. Cover the container. Leave it in a well-lit place and proceed as above to check for germination, then transfer sprouted seeds to pots.

The bottle keeps the paper towels moist, although it's probably overkill, since there is so little evaporation anyway inside the closed plastic container. This definitely feels more "mad scientist" than just some paper towels in a bag!

### Read all about it: Use your newspapers

This is my favorite seed starting method. You can make pots for almost free, from newspapers, some glue, and a cylindrical form. Cut long, narrow strips and wrap them around the cylindrical form, with about 1/4 or 1/3 of the length sticking out past the bottom of the form.

Add some glue on the end to secure it. (This is optional, but it seems to help it stay together and be more stable, especially when your pots are small).

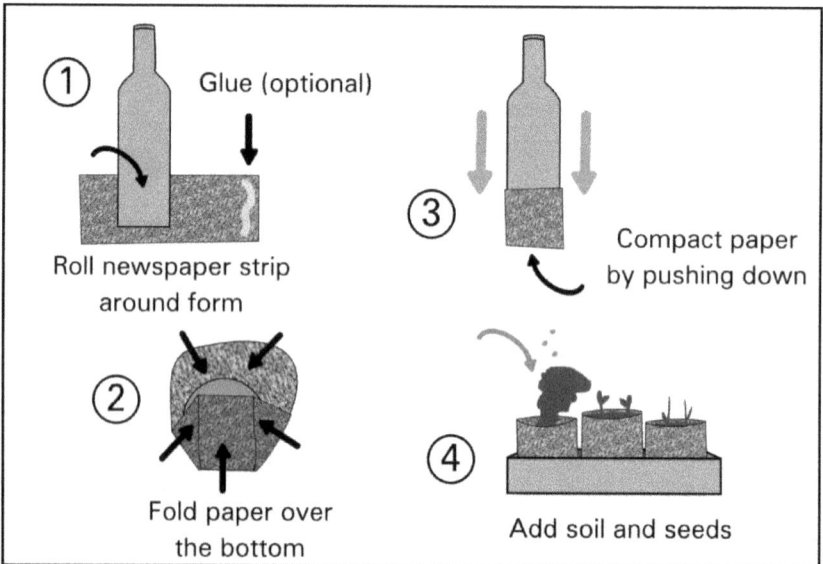

Fold the overhanging paper over the form towards the center, to create the bottom of the pot. Press the form down securely on a table top or something solid, to squeeze the newspapers in firmly.

When the glue dries, you can add growing medium and plant your seeds in them. Put several of them inside some sort of container with high sides, to help keep them from falling over. We like to use old 5-gallon bucket bottoms. When the plastic gets old and brittle, the tops often break off. This is a good way to use what is left.

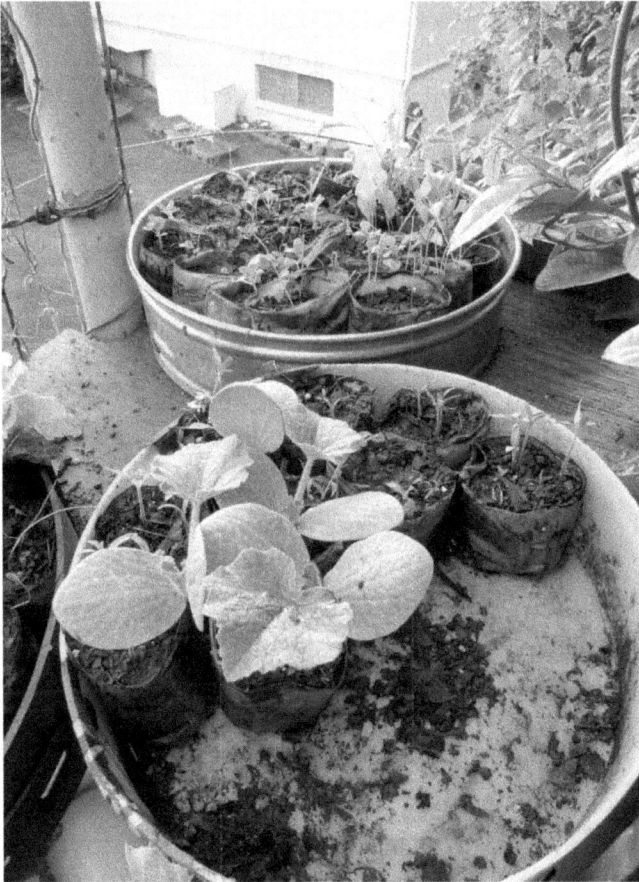

The newspaper absorbs moisture, helping the seeds to germinate. And because it's biodegradable, you can plant the entire thing, pot and all, when you transplant into the garden.

However, the roots tend to grow between the folds of paper at the bottom of the pot. Also, the layers of newspaper can be a bit hard to penetrate, and they dry out and get stiff and do not break down readily. So I like to carefully peel away as much of the pot as I can when transplanting, leaving some pieces of the newspaper bottom, if the roots of the seedling are growing through them.

You can use an empty jar or bottle as your form. A wine bottle with a depression in the bottom helps to allow you to smash the paper in it. You can buy a commercial form, make one out of PVC pipe, or if you turn wood or know a woodturner, you can make your own. There are links to online information at the end of this book.

## Dry farming seed starting

In dry and sandier soils, plant seeds as deep as possible. The theory behind this is because, in desert and arid climates, moisture is stored in the soil at a deep level. By planting deeply, you take advantage of that stored moisture, which you wouldn't even reach if planted at the normal recommended package planting depths.

Planting deeply also encourages deep rooting, which leads to heartier, more drought-resistant plants. Seed can more easily push through sandy, loose soils than compacted clays, so planting deeper is fine.

What is a recommended depth? Start at 4 inches (10 cm) and experiment with going as deep as 8 inches (20 cm). Plant in a hole in the bottom of a furrow. The furrow helps to channel any available moisture down to the seed, and it also acts as a buffer against some of the wind.

# CHAPTER 8

## It's Not What You Do, It's How You Do It: Water-Saving Garden Types

You might be familiar with only the traditional method of growing crops, in long rows with wide spaces between them. But this method was developed for mechanized agriculture, and it's not the most efficient or even recommended in a home garden. Here are some other alternatives to consider.

### Not just for breakfast

If you pour syrup on a waffle, the syrup will pool in the little squares, because the raised bits between them create natural barriers. In the same way, grids of rectangles and squares can be created in the ground, with soil berms (walls) between them. When it rains, the moisture stays inside the walls, and none is wasted by runoff.

Create square planting areas 2 feet (61 cm) across, bordered by berms several inches (about 6 cm) high, made from unamended soil. You could also use rocks as borders.

Mulch the growing area with gravel, sand, or rock, at least 2-3 inches (5-7.5 cm) deep. Gravel-sized mulch is most effective, because all of the water will flow through it, into the soil below, reducing runoff. The gravel also captures condensation that occurs when temperatures rise, and drips that moisture around the rocks and down, into the soil.

## Square foot gardening

This system was made popular by Mel Bartholomew, author of
the book by the same name. It lays out plants in areas that are
all one foot (30 cm) square.

Smaller plants, such as carrots, can be spaced so there are 16
plants in one square. Medium plants, like beets, are planted
nine to a square. Larger plants, such as lettuce, are planted four
to a square. And very large plants, such as cabbages and
tomatoes, take an entire square per plant.

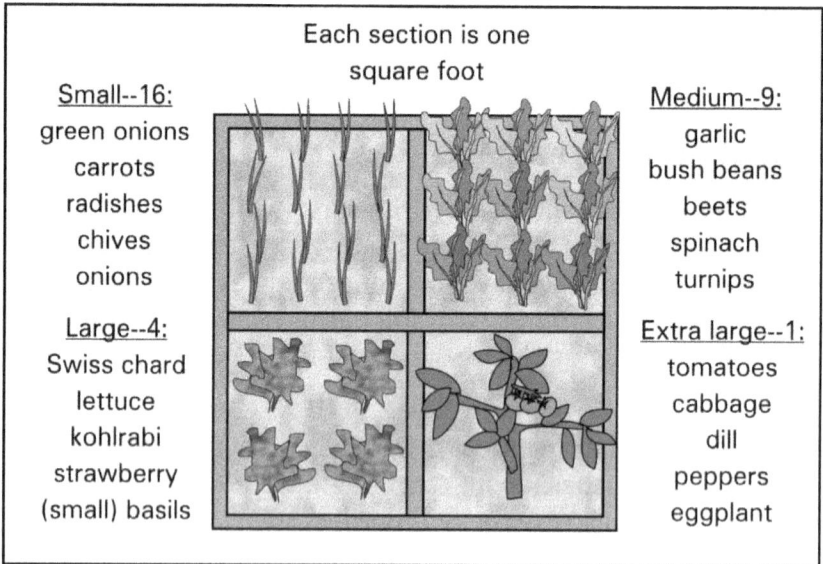

Planting this way ensures that there is very little room for
weeds to compete for space and nutrients, and it makes
maximum use of your garden space. When plants are ready to
be pulled, you have seedlings of a different type of vegetable
ready to be planted in the same square, maximizing harvest
from your growing season.

This rotates crops, since no type of plant is put into the same
spot twice. Doing so reduces the spread of soil-borne diseases.

## Lasagna gardening: In-place layering

Instead of building a compost pile in a separate location, you put organic materials into the soil where you will later be gardening, wetting them as you go. After six to twelve months, the material should have broken down naturally, and you can plant there.

Some people do this over a layer of cardboard or several thicknesses of newspaper, to prevent weeds from coming up. You can also put the material down, then cover all of it with a layer of finished compost or soil, and plant into that. Eventually, the layers below break down, providing nutrients.

## Subversive designs: Sub-irrigated planters

If plants have a constant need for water, why not provide a constant supply? Sub-irrigated planters and systems put water in a below-crop chamber. Plant roots can dip into the moisture and use as much of it as they want, whenever they want.

You can buy commercially-made planters, or make your own. There are many different homemade systems being tested and developed by gardeners, including those that use kiddie pools, rain gutters, or large trays to hold water reserves.

One problem is that having an open water source is the perfect breeding ground for mosquitoes. Although not much of a problem in North America, malaria--which is spread by mosquitoes--still kills many people worldwide. And mosquitoes spread other diseases, such as Dengue Fever, West Nile Virus, various forms of encephalitis, and heartworm in dogs.

For this reason, I suggest you use only sub-irrigation systems that are closed and do not allow standing water where mosquitoes can breed. There are hybrid systems being tested that hold water below ground, with pipes connecting growing containers. Or use a system similar to the one I will explain below, which has a covered water section.

There are also multiple designs using two containers, such as buckets, or the top and bottom of an empty soda bottle, to hold the growing medium and plant above, separated from the reservoir below. Because the moisture is far below the plants, and gravity won't carry it upwards, you need a way to wick it to the growing medium. There it can move into the plant root zone, to be taken up by the plant and used. Eventually, your plant roots may grow long enough to reach that reservoir. In the meantime, however, you need something as a wick.

You can try using thread or string, or a strip of absorbent fabric, such as an old t-shirt or towel. But because anything cotton is biodegradable, these wicks can degrade fast and will need to be replaced often. People have had success using polyester and other synthetic materials for wicks, which last longer. You will have to experiment to see what is easily obtainable in your area and works well.

One of the drawbacks to these systems is their heavy reliance on wicking potting soils and peat moss-based growing substrates, which also help hold moisture and pull it upwards. Peat moss is a non-renewable resource. It has taken hundreds of years for the moss to grow, and it provides an important role in its ecosystem. The widespread use of peat moss for gardening is causing degradation and environmental damage, and it needs to stop, before we see widespread desertification in the bogs too.

Many systems use potting soil, which is often a sterile medium, devoid of all life, with added chemical fertilizers and amendments. While these may give you good results in the short term, they are not natural parts of a healthy ecosystem, and you will forever be reliant on them for good production.

End your reliance on those artificial or non-renewable garden amendments and fertilizers. Instead, please consider using more renewable materials, such as coconut coir in place of peat moss, and incorporating lots of organic materials, such as compost and wood chips, which help retain moisture and encourage healthy microbial growth, leading to a long-term, productive, living soil.

Using synthetic chemicals and potting soil actually reduces the long-term fertility of the soil. The fertilizers kill microbes in the soil, including mycorrhizal fungi. And potting soil, once it gets completely dry, is very difficult to return to a state where it will absorb moisture again.

I'm including links at the end of the book, if you want to check out some of these sub-irrigation ideas. Please consider ways to use renewable materials in these systems, instead of the commercial, synthetic, and non-renewable ones that most of them rely on.

If you do use potting mixes, choose those without added chemical fertilizers, and add your own organic amendments, such as compost, kelp and alfalfa. I know I keep repeating the message to choose organic materials over synthetics. I know that it's too easy to be suckered into the lush, easy growth that you get from synthetic products.

But unless you consciously choose to build soil that is healthy and fertile, you can mindlessly keep using the chemicals. That is exactly why we are in trouble these days.

Big-company hybrid seeds, chemical fertilizers and materials, and mechanized methods have depleted the soil and created produce that relies on them. If you continue to use these products, you will be dependent on them, too.

The alternative is to build soil that is naturally productive and fertile. But this takes time, and you need to add a lot of organic material in order to see results. Most people want the quick, easy way, regardless of the long-term effects.

Please be conscious and make choices that benefit the long-term productivity of the soil, not the short-term showiness. Our planet, and our own lives, depend on us making wiser choices.

## In-place, self-watering  beds and containers

Some gardeners have created sub-irrigated spaces in the ground by putting down plastic sheeting and creating a water-holding chamber under their in-ground crops.  Water is pumped through pipes or poured down tubing to the underground chamber.  This way they can incorporate compost and other soil amendments, without relying on potting soil or peat moss.

Some gardeners have been able to create sub-irrigated planters in containers, using mostly renewable, organic matter.  Gravel, broken pots, empty plastic bottles, or irrigation drainage pipe is placed in the bottom of a water-holding container, to create a void for the water.  Above that, a barrier of weed landscaping fabric acts to prevent the soil from settling to the bottom and clogging the irrigation pipe, filling the reservoir, or draining away.

On top of that, sand is added to wick the moisture upwards toward the growing medium.  Above that, organic material is added, which will break down over time and retain moisture.  Topping it all off is a growing medium rich in compost or other organic material.  Plants are added and mulched.

A drainage portal is created so that excess water can drain out, preventing waterlogging of the soil.  Keep the drain below the level of any organic material.  Otherwise, you'll get a stinky swamp smell, from organic material decomposing in water.

Water is added to the holding chamber via a filling tube.  Moisture is wicked upwards by the gravel and sand, where it is retained in the organic material in the soil.

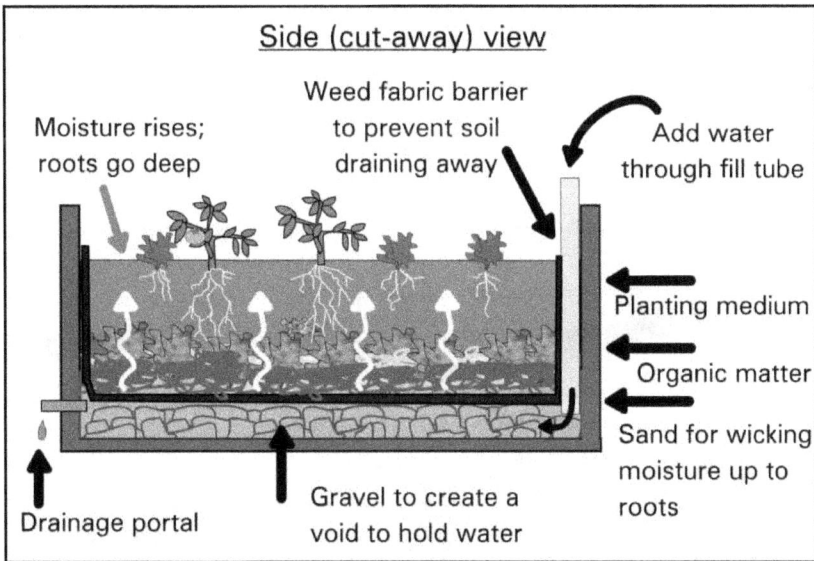

Side (cut-away) view

Weed fabric barrier
Moisture rises;          to prevent soil          Add water
roots go deep            draining away            through fill tube

Planting medium

Organic matter

Sand for wicking
moisture up to
roots

Drainage portal          Gravel to create a
                         void to hold water

Plant roots grow down, looking for moisture. They find and absorb it whenever they want, leading to increased production and tremendous growth. You use very little water this way, because there is almost nothing wasted.

## Soda bottle self-waterers

If you think you don't have the time, money, or space to grow anything, think again. Self-irrigating planters can be made with bottles that are going to be thrown away. All you need is a well-lit window sill or some indoor grow lights, and you can grow something. Stick to herbs, leafy greens, and lettuce if you have low light levels and a small space. You'll have delicious salads that will get you itching to grow more.

Take an empty plastic beverage bottle. Cut it into two pieces about halfway down.

Take a strip of old flannel, t-shirt, or towel and tie it into a knot. Remove the bottle cap. Drop the long end through the hole in the top of the bottle.

Add growing medium to the top of the bottle (turned upside down).  Pack it in well in the neck of the bottle, around the wick. Add seeds or a transplant.

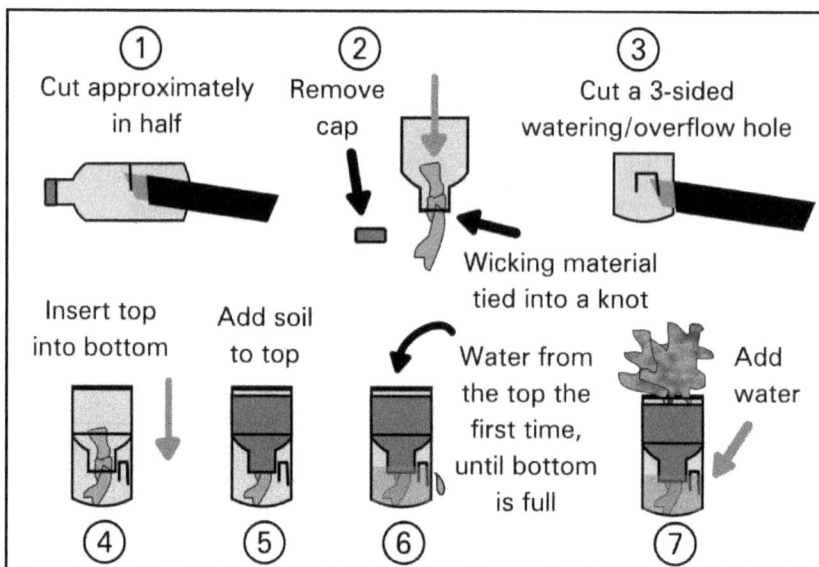

If you decide to use your own soil or compost mix as the growing medium, check it after a couple days to be sure it is wicking and retaining enough moisture. Poke your finger down into it. The medium should be moist, not dry. You may need to add moisture-retaining materials, such as woodchips, coconut coir, or peat moss, if it is not retaining moisture.

Place the top into the bottom of the bottle. If it won't fit easily, you can cut short, vertical slits around the top edge of the bottom section of the bottle. They will fan open just enough to allow the top to fit in.

If your bottle has a narrow "waist" to it, you may need to trim away that center section altogether. Then the top should fit, or cut vertical slits in the bottom section, to allow it to.

Water from the top the first time you use it.  Water until the bottom chamber is full.

The fabric will wick moisture up from the chamber below and moisten the growing medium. Natural fabrics, such as cotton, will break down eventually, so you may opt to use polyester or other synthetic fabric, such as weed barrier, shade cloth, or a piece of a woven reusable shopping bag, instead. You may need to experiment to see what you have that will work.

When the water gets low, refill it by adding water through the filling/overflow window you made. You can push the piece of plastic inwards, to give you more room for a watering spout. You could also just pull the whole top section out of the bottom section, add water, then reassemble.

Instead of the fabric, paper can be your wicking agent. Use a paper towel, folded into a short, tight roll, which is stuck into another paper towel, which is molded around the bottom of the towel roll and left flared around the inside edge of the top bottle. Or use the same sort of shape with newspaper. The papers will absorb water, draw it upwards, and wet the growing medium.

## Go shopping for grow bags

This is a similar idea to the sub-irrigation planters, but in a simplified form. Plants are grown in fabric pouches or bags, which are placed in, or suspended over, a tray or other container with water in it.

You can sew your own bags from weed-barrier cloth sold in garden centers, or use already-made fabric shopping bags. These can be purchased, or you can use what you have, if you have a large supply from shopping.

Depending on the size and shape of the bags, they may not stand up by themselves too well and may need to be placed in a container that helps support them. You may have to fiddle with the size and shape of the bags if you sew them yourself, in order to get something more sturdy.

For irrigating, you can rest the bags on plastic lids, with holes cut in the lids, so the plant roots go down into the water in a trough below. Or just stand them in a container with water in the bottom. Make sure the container has a drainage hole partway up the side, so the plant does not drown.

Sunlight breaks down the fabric of these bags, so they will eventually fall apart. Because they are not biodegradable, you end up with wasted plastic bits that go into a landfill. Walmart shopping bags are reported to be more resistant to breakdown from sunlight than other fabrics.

I've tried this method using regular compost, but I wasn't sure if I could get wicking action, so I just kept watering from above. The excess water was in the bottom of the tub where the bags were.

A few things I didn't like were that the bags tended to be somewhat floppy, so they did not stand upright well and needed to lean on each other and be in a container with high sides, to support them. Another problem is that slugs tend to multiply and hang out between and under the bags, which led to an overpopulation that destroyed the crops. Mosquitoes bred in the collected water. The fabric (I used weed barrier cloth) broke down, so the bags are falling apart, and I can't reuse them. So for me, this method hasn't worked well.

### Air pruning/sub-irrigation hybrids

You can experiment with air pruning (see the end of Chapter 10) and sub-irrigation by using plastic pots with multiple small holes drilled in the sides. This will air-prune the roots and create more vigor. Line them with weed-barrier landscape fabric. This will hold the growing medium in.

Construct the rest of your sub-irrigation system normally. I have yet to try air pruning methods, but some gardeners are getting great results.

## The ghetto gardens

Sack or bag gardens are being used in parts of Africa, especially where there is no good soil because of rocks, or in the cities, where people have no land and very little money. They make use of what would normally be thrown away.

Potatoes, rice, and other dry crops are sold in large plastic bags and are easy to obtain. The bags are used as containers, which can be placed on the ground.

Roll the top of the bag down around the outside until it is about one foot (30 cm) from the bottom. Place the bag where you want it to end up permanently.

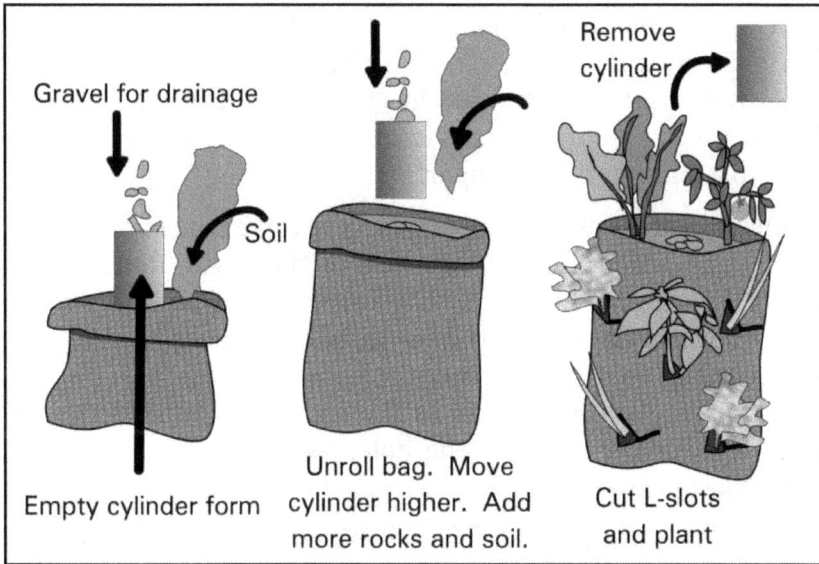

Gravel for drainage

Soil

Remove cylinder

Empty cylinder form

Unroll bag. Move cylinder higher. Add more rocks and soil.

Cut L-slots and plant

Make a small-diameter, tall cylinder out of a coffee can with both ends cut out, a length of wide PVC pipe, or something else sturdy. Place the cylinder in the center of the bag.

Add rocks or pea gravel to the cylinder about 2/3 of the way up to the top. Add growing medium around the cylinder, filling up the bag.

As you get near the top, unroll the edges of the bag to make it taller, and carefully lift the cylinder up, leaving the rocks in place.  Basically, you are trying to create a central column of rocks, which helps to stabilize the bag, increase drainage and keep the plants' roots cool, inside a bag full of growing medium.  Think of the rocks like where the hole in a doughnut would be.

Continue adding rocks, and soil, unrolling the top of the bag and pulling up the cylinder, until you have filled the entire bag.  Stop when you have about 2-3 inches (5-7.5 cm) left at the top of the bag.  That is so the soil will not flow over the top rim of the bag and fall out when you water or plant in it.  Remove your cylinder and use it when making your next bag.

You may need to add some supports to the bag to keep it upright and stable.  You can do so by tying it to three or four long sticks, which reach from the ground to above the top of the bag, spaced around the outside of the bag.  Or tie or wire the bags to a fence or other supports.

To plant, add seeds for tall plants to the top of the bag.  Smaller plants are added around the sides of the bag.  Cut L-shaped slices through the plastic with a knife, poke a hole in the soil with your finger, and add the seedlings.  If you need support for the seedling so it doesn't droop and fall out, cut half a plastic cup (cut lengthwise), or half of the top of a plastic bottle, and stick the narrow end into the hole, so it forms a cup-shaped, shelf-like support.

This method works best for cut-and-come-again leafy greens such as kale, collards, leaf lettuce, and Swiss chard.  You can pick the outer leaves, and the plant will continue to grow, producing food over a long period of time.  Strawberries or green onions, as well as smaller herbs, such as thyme, rosemary, or chives, also do well along the sides.

## Aquaponics and Pee-ponics

These systems use nutrients in the water as fertilizer, and many systems do away with soil or any growing medium whatsoever. These are beyond the scope of this book, but I wanted to mention them in case they might be of interest to you.

Aquaponics basically uses a tank with fish in it. You feed the fish, they poop into the water, and the water is used to water the plants. Fish excrement acts as fertilizer.

Pee-ponics uses human urine instead of the fish poop. Diluted human urine is an excellent source of nitrogen.

Both of these are forms of hydroponics, which uses chemical fertilizers dissolved in water as the source of nutrients for plants.

## Don't throw it out: Bottle tower and PVC pipe gardens

Both these designs use the same principle: Water into the top of a column, and the water filters down, feeding plants along the way. Any leftover moisture is collected at the bottom and reused by pouring it back in at the top.

The towers can be connected to a drip irrigation system, which is fed by a rain- or water-catchment system. Make sure the bottom-most section or end cap has holes for drainage, so that the roots at the very bottom do not end up drowning in waterlogged, airless soil or growing medium.

Both of these will need to be attached to some sort of frame, such as a pole, fence, wall, or a pillar made of wire mesh-- anything that will hold it upright and help support the weight.

One of the benefits of vertical gardening is that you can use discarded material that might otherwise end up in a landfill. Vertical gardening also takes up less room on the ground, so it works well for people with a limited amount of space. These can be installed on a patio or next to a house, for example, where you would not normally have enough room to grow things in the ground or large containers.

Some people have concerns that the plastic may leach harmful chemicals when heated by the sun, or when in contact with the growing medium long-term. BPA, Bisphenol A, is one of the chemicals of concern. It's in some plastics and epoxy resins used in the lining of metal cans and bottle tops. It may leach out and affect the brain and behavior of fetuses, infants, and children. [6]

Another drawback is that you are limited to somewhat smaller plants and herbs in this system.

## Bottle tower garden

There are many different designs using discarded plastic 1- or 2-liter soft drink or beverage bottles, but here is one of them. Cut the bottoms off all bottles. The caps are removed from all but the bottom and top bottles, which are stacked, upside-down, one on top of the other, much like when you built a tower of blocks as a child. (Then your baby brother or sister came stomping by and knocked the whole thing down. Grr!)

Drill two drainage holes about 2 inches (5 cm) up from the very bottom, in the bottom bottle, to allow for excess water to drain off. Drill a hole in the cap of the top bottle, and insert it into a second bottle which is empty, and is used like a funnel.

Place the top bottle and the funnel on top of the remaining bottles, which are all filled with growing medium. Cut a three-

---

[6] National Institutes of Health, U.S. Department of Health and Human Services, National Institute of Environmental Health Sciences, https://www.niehs.nih.gov/health/topics/agents/sya-bpa/ (accessed April 24, 2014).

sided window out of the sides of those bottles, for planting. Add a seedling in each, and water from the top.

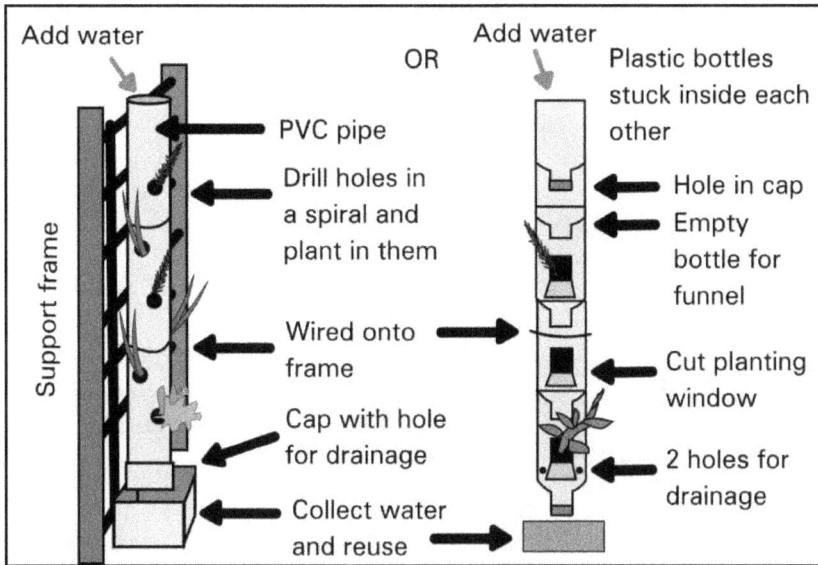

## PVC garden

Use a length of PVC pipe with a cap on the bottom end. Drill a hole in the end cap or on the sides of the pipe just above the end cap, to allow for drainage.

Drill holes in a spiral pattern around the sides of the PVC pipe. Fill the entire thing with growing medium and insert seedlings into the holes. Water from the top and collect the excess moisture at the bottom, to be reused.

## The pizza and pie combo

In Africa, where drought is threatening to cut off the food supply for many people, keyhole gardening is coming to the rescue. The gardens are designed to use any available waste material and create a compact, water-efficient, sustainable garden.

It is like a combination of compost pile and garden plot, all in one compact, round unit.  Picture a pizza, or a pie (are you in the mood for savory or sweet?) with one slice missing.  That is the keyhole shape to aim for.

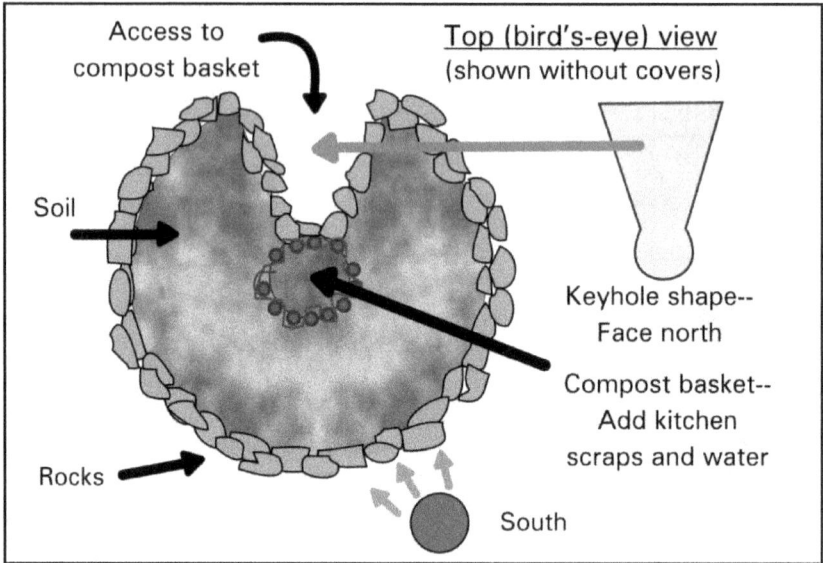

The outside is made of bricks, stone, clay, and in modern settings, beer or wine bottles set in cement.  In the middle, a small, tall tube is formed using wire mesh or sticks and string.

You put compost material, including manure, straw, wood ash, shredded newspaper, and kitchen scraps, into the center compost "basket" area, and water it down well.  The rest of the garden is also filled with waste material, including sticks, bones, old telephone books, cardboard, straw, rusty cans, and other organic scraps.  Use something in the bottom layer that will help with drainage, such as broken terra cotta pots, sticks, or stones.

On top of all that, you put a thick layer of compost or soil that is ready for planting.  Mound it higher in the center, so that moisture can run out from the basket towards the walls.

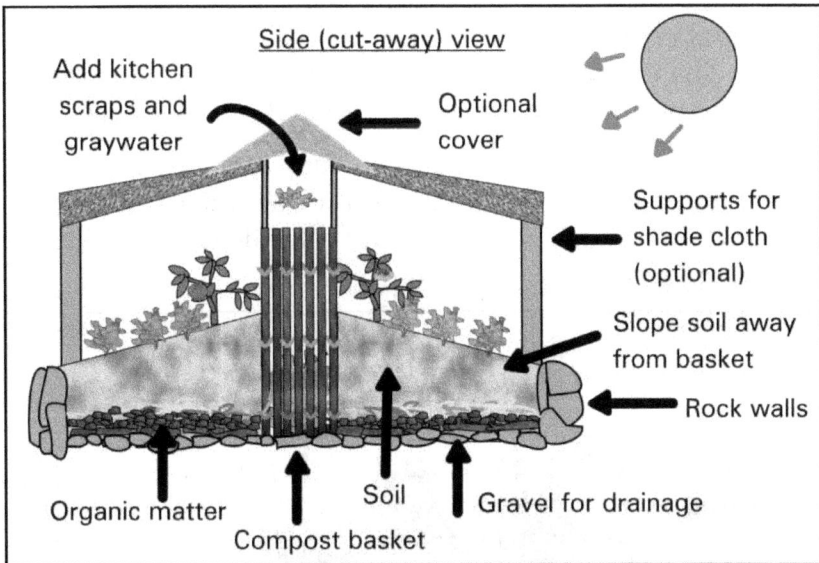

Side (cut-away) view

Add kitchen scraps and graywater

Optional cover

Supports for shade cloth (optional)

Slope soil away from basket

Rock walls

Organic matter

Soil

Compost basket

Gravel for drainage

Place seedlings in the outer area and water well. As you get more kitchen scraps and vegetable peels, etc., you add them into the center compost "basket." Moisture from this central column forces the plant roots to go deeper into the soil, searching for moisture, which helps create more hardy plants that are able to withstand lower water levels more easily.

You can add a roof to the center section, to help prevent evaporation in hot weather. Or a frame which can support shade fabric, to reduce sun in the summer. It can then be used with plastic sheeting to create a greenhouse in cooler weather.

## Going in circles:  Spiral garden

This garden is extremely convenient when planted close to your kitchen. You can go outside and snip something for your soup, stew pot, or salad whenever you want. You get spoiled having fresh herbs whenever you need them. And you save a lot of money, too.

The spiral creates a few different microclimates in a compact
space.  The center section, which is higher than the outsides,
will be for plants that prefer more heat and better drainage.

You can add different soil mixtures, such as more or less sand,
to different areas of the spiral, or just use the same compost and
soil mixture throughout.  Water will filter down and collect in
the bottom sections.

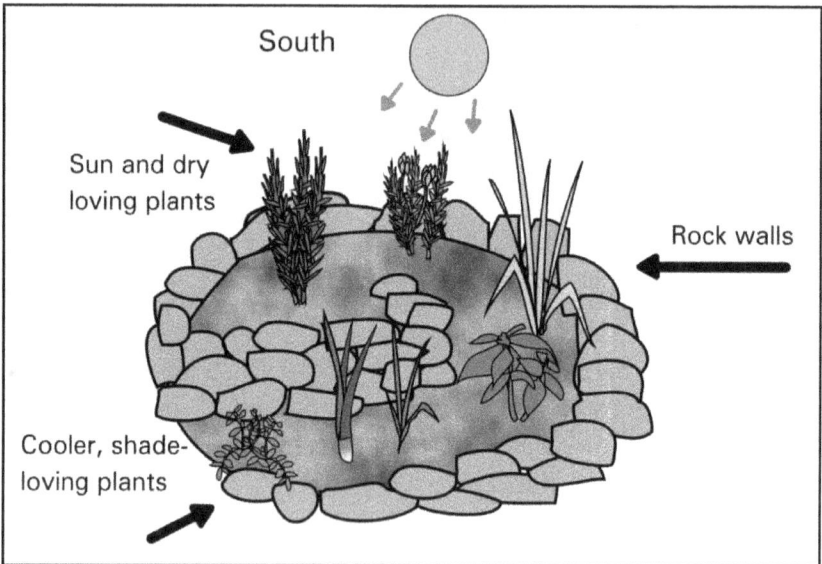

To create the garden, mark out your spiral shape about 6 feet (2
meters) in diameter and 2-3 feet (60-100 cm) high.  Use rocks or
bricks to create a wall to hold soil in.  The center section, which
is highest, will need something to increase drainage on the
bottom and fill up space, topped with a planting mix.  You can
use old broken concrete, branches, wood chips, gravel, or
broken pots as filler.

Fill the top with herbs that like more sun and better drainage,
the bottom with plants that like less sun and more moisture,
and the middle with those that like in-between conditions.  You
can fill in open spaces with kale, nasturtium, and calendula.

Plant those things that need more sun on the south-facing sections of the spiral, since about one half of the spiral will get sun, and the other half will get more shade.

Here are some suggested plants for the different areas:

***Top zone:*** rosemary, oregano, sage, thyme, marjoram, lavender

***Middle zone:*** sorrel, parsley, lemon balm, lemongrass, tarragon, basil, arugula

***Bottom zone:*** mints, cilantro, chives, green onions, dill, pennyroyal, chamomile

# CHAPTER 9

## Go Big if You Can: Modifying Your Landscape

Clearly the message to be learned, from the real-world examples we looked at earlier, is that if you want permanent, lasting change to your area, you need to make permanent, lasting change to your area. Of course, this is only possible when you own the land you live on or are allowed to make changes, and you have the resources and ability to do so.

But if you're interested, here are a few ways that can really make a difference. Again, anything you do will have different results depending on your location and the weather patterns you experience there.

One way to increase your odds of success is by observation. Take a walk around your area and see what kinds of plants are doing well, especially in areas where there is no human care involved. That's a good way to find out what sorts of wild herbs, flowers, trees, shrubs, and plants can grow easily with little care on your part.

Next, look at what nature is doing, and see if you find any patterns. For example, are certain plants growing in clumps? Are any of them near formations of rocks, or in depressions? Are any plants always found together?

By observing what works well in your area, you may be able to discern important bits of information that others have missed. Nature has infinite wisdom, and those who can figure it out are so much the wiser. When we find ways to work with nature, such as harnessing the power from the sun or wind, or taking advantage of natural rainfall patterns, we can benefit without causing harm.

## Bury the evidence

Hugelkultur is an efficient way to use up excess tree trimmings, logs, and branches on your property and turn them into water-holding reservoirs for your plants. The word in German translates to "mound culture," because when you build them above ground, you form mounded shapes.

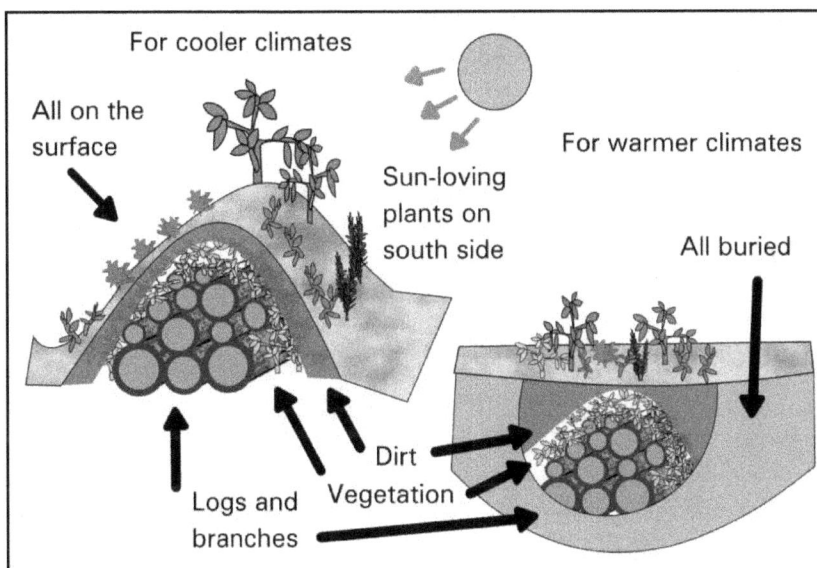

The basic recipe is very simple. Place logs in an area where you want to grow something, cover it with soil and any extra organic material, and plant in it. As the logs and branches break down, they provide even more fertility for your plants.

In the meantime, however, they act like sponges. If you use freshly cut trees, they are already loaded with water. If you use older wood, the decomposing fibers hold lots of moisture, making it available to your plants.

For best results, use smaller things like leaves and straw to fill in the voids between logs. Add some material high in nitrogen, such as green leaves or grass clippings, chicken manure, or human urine.

If you build over an area with existing grass, cut the sod off the top, then lay it, face down, over the top of the logs.  This will provide nitrogen and prevent caving in, by helping to fill in the holes between the larger logs.

Press everything down when you're done, if you do this in a mound, so it holds together.  Water it well, and you can add something like straw or leaves on top to act as mulch.  You can also "pin" the mulch into the sides with long sticks placed horizontally, held into the mound by short sticks made from forked branches.

Avoid using walnut tree logs or branches, which have a naturally-occurring chemical that is toxic to many other plants.  It's like putting pesticides in the soil, then trying to grow in it.

Some people have found that they need to water very little, to not at all, especially once the plants are established.  But the shape of the hugelkultur mound seems to make a big difference.

In colder climates, making mounds, sometimes as high as 6-7 feet (about 2 meters) seems to work the best.  There is usually some settling and shrinking that occurs as the wood breaks down.  Sun-loving plants can be positioned on the south-facing sides of the mound.

In warmer climates, however, or windier ones, tall mounds dry out, and the soil blows away.  So small mounds or underground mounds are preferred.

Usually trees or other large plants, such as sunflowers, corn, beans, peas, and tomatoes are positioned at the top, and different plants are mixed together along the sides of the mound.

Be sure to plant a wide variety, all mixed up together.  If you grow by sowing seeds, overseed.  In other words, plant more seeds than you know you'll need, so you'll have lush growth.  Be sure to add some herbs or flowers that will attract beneficial insects and bees, for pest control and pollination.

You will definitely want to water well the first year if you are using new wood which has not yet broken down, because it won't be spongy enough to hold more moisture, yet it already contains some, which will get filtered into the surrounding soil.

Both types of mound will tend to do better over time. The first year you will probably get okay results, and years afterwards will improve.

The simplicity of the method, and its adaptability, make it worth trying if you have the chance to. It's certainly cheaper than paying to have tree trimmings hauled to a landfill or greenwaste facility. And you've already learned how valuable organic material, with its nutrient- and moisture-providing capability, is to plant growth.

(By the way, if you cut or trim a tree and have usable wood that you'd rather see gets made into something, consider contacting your local woodworking or woodturning club, or a college that offers woodworking classes. They will often gladly take your wood, and you will know it is getting made into useful objects, instead of just getting thrown away, or rotting somewhere. Usable wood is firm, not rotted or punky, and free from bugs or nails. You could also donate the larger stump pieces and put just the smaller leaves and branches into a hugelkultur mound).

## Water Engineering

If you have a large amount of property that you own or can make changes to, the most efficient way to change the way your landscape uses and holds water is to modify and design it so that the flow of water is slowed, spread throughout the area, and stays there.

All of the remaining methods we'll look at involve long-term changes to your property and must be carefully designed and implemented. The following information in this chapter is provided just as an overview. DO NOT attempt to implement any of these changes without further information.  See the Learn More section at the end of the book for resources.

# Basic principles

### Stay away from pipes

Be sure any area you plan to dig in is free from pipes or other underground structures.

### Start at the top

You want to start at the highest point of your property and work your way down to the lowest point.  Making changes up high, where any water is moving slowly, is easier to do and more likely to get results, than any changes lower, or where the flow of water is large or fast.

### Spread the water around

You want water to move in a broad area, rather than flowing in a narrow segment.  This is best accomplished by spreading your planting around, rather than keeping it in one area.

### Stay away from foundations

You need to be sure any of these changes are at least 10 feet (3 meters) away from a building's foundation.  Otherwise, you can weaken the structure and possibly cause harm or destruction.

### Start small

Begin by making small changes.

### Always plan an overflow route

In a large storm, excess rainwater can cause flooding or erosion. You need to have a plan for what happens to any water that is not absorbed by your landscape as it stands.  Some people create ponds on their property to handle the overflow.

## Observe and make changes

Start by observing what happens already when it rains or storms. Look for patterns of runoff and erosion. See where plants are already thriving, and study why that may be so. Apply your observations to any changes you make, and modify them to incorporate new knowledge. Experiment (carefully!) and learn from your experience.

## Consult an expert

I do not even pretend to be an expert when it comes to landscape modifications. Consult a qualified professional when necessary or if you are in doubt about anything.

Check the resources at the back of the book for my recommended reading if you plan to implement any of the following modifications. The information provided here is NOT meant to be a how-to guide. It is just to introduce you to what is possible. These methods can cause flooding and destruction, so you need to be knowledgeable before you attempt to use any of them. Do your homework and learn about these techniques if you plan to try them.

# Swales

Swales are ditches that are dug on contour with the land. They provide catchment for natural rainfall and water. When it rains, water is channeled into the swale and then percolates slowly into the area just below it. Swales act to slow or stop water that might otherwise speed down a hill (even a very mild slope) and can then be used to irrigate an area far from other water sources.

Just like a ball rolling down a hill will pick up speed as it goes along, so will water. So it's most effective to start at the highest point on your property that you can work, and continue to add more swales further downhill. The steeper your land, and the more rain washes down it, the more closely together and more frequent your swales should be.

It's the same principle as is used in terraced fields. I'm sure you've seen images of terraced rice paddies or other fields in mountains, which look like stairs. You're using that same principle, but the swales are acting like stairs, allowing water to "step" down instead of "rolling."

Do not put swales within 10 feet (3 meters) of a wall or foundation. They are to be used on slopes of 3:1 gradient or less. That means for every 3 units of measure (such as feet or meters), there is a drop of 1 unit or less. For gradients that are steeper than that, you will need to use retaining walls and terraces.

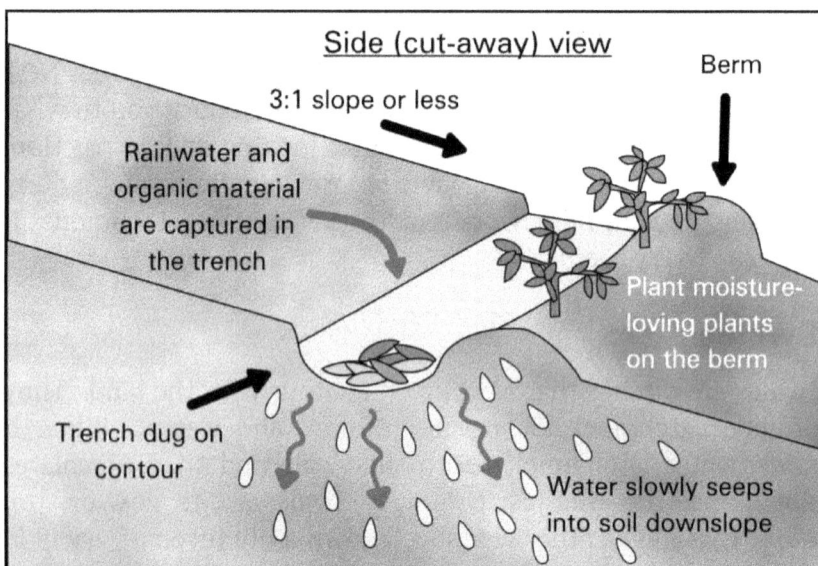

Side (cut-away) view
Berm
3:1 slope or less
Rainwater and organic material are captured in the trench
Plant moisture-loving plants on the berm
Trench dug on contour
Water slowly seeps into soil downslope

Swales are dug on contour lines, imaginary horizontal lines that are level and follow the natural contours of the earth. You cannot guess at contour lines. They must be measured and marked using a homemade A-frame tool.

To make an A-frame tool, connect two equal-length pieces of 2 x 4, poles, or wood into the top of an A shape. Attach a crosspiece so that both ends are the same distance from the bottom ends of the side (leg) pieces.

The height of the A-frame should be about as tall as you are, between 5 and 6 feet (0.3-1.8 meters). The legs should be at least 3 feet (0.9 meters) apart.

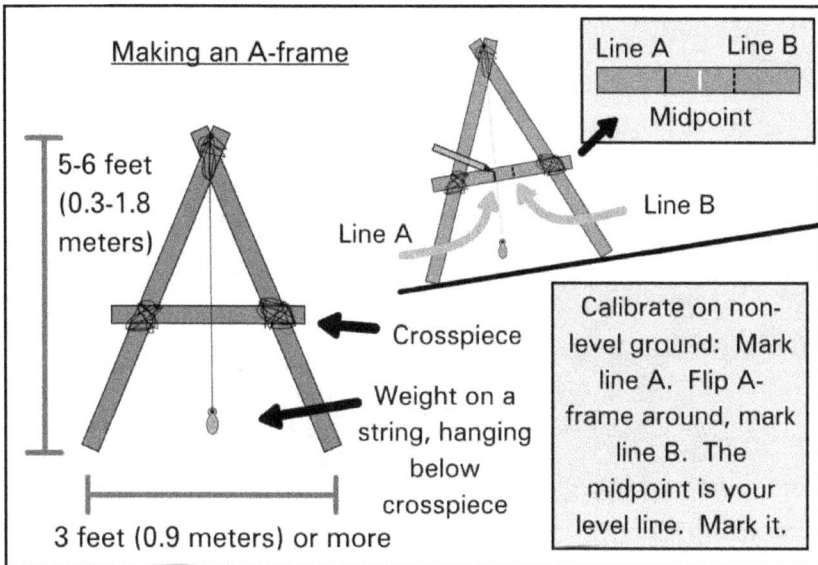

Making an A-frame

5-6 feet (0.3-1.8 meters)

Line A

Line B

Line A     Line B

Midpoint

Crosspiece

Weight on a string, hanging below crosspiece

3 feet (0.9 meters) or more

Calibrate on non-level ground: Mark line A. Flip A-frame around, mark line B. The midpoint is your level line. Mark it.

You have two choices for making the A frame work as a level. One option is to attach a spirit level to the crosspiece.

The second option is to hang a string from the top of the A, with a weight or plumb bob at the end, which hangs lower than the crosspiece. You will need to calibrate this by placing the A frame on non-level ground, then marking a vertical line (line A) where the string crosses on the crosspiece.

Flip the A-frame around, then mark (line B) on the opposite side where the string crosses on the crosspiece. Measure the exact center between those two lines, your midpoint. Mark it. When you place the A-frame on level ground, the string will fall over your midpoint line.

To use your A-frame, place the two legs on your property where you want to begin your contour line. Move one leg until you are level. Place a flag or stake in the ground to mark the position of both legs.

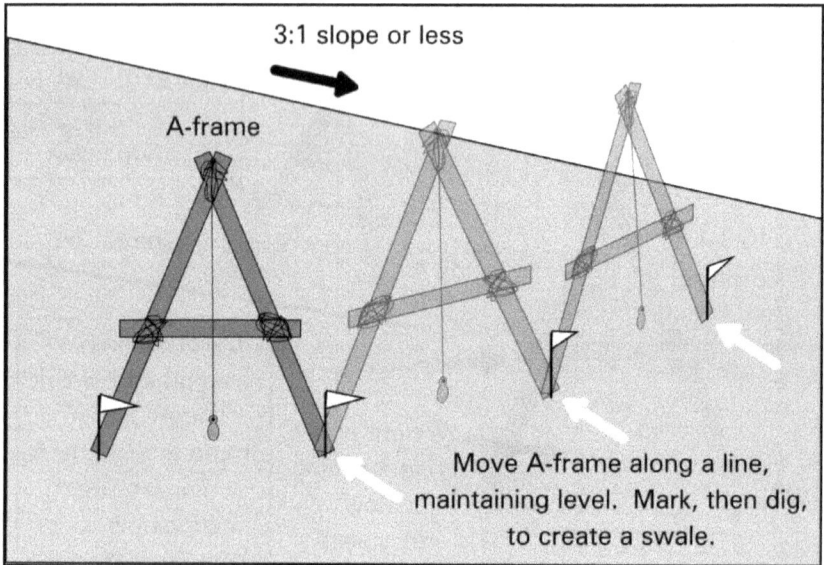

3:1 slope or less

A-frame

Move A-frame along a line, maintaining level. Mark, then dig, to create a swale.

Move over so the first leg is where the second just was, and then move the second leg around, until you get a level reading. Add another stake or flag at the bottom of the second leg.

Repeat this procedure until you have mapped out your contour line or lines. Dig a trench along your contour line that is approximately 1 foot (0.3 meters) deep by three feet (0.9 meter) wide. Place the soil you remove on the lower side of the trench, to create your berm.

Once you think the trench is fairly level, put a garden hose in it and flood the area. You will see where there are high spots that need to be dug out more.

Fill the trench with tree trimmings topped by straw, sawdust, or mulch. You can use the berm as a planting area by mounding it with compost and other organic material and planting, then mulching on it. Or use it for a pathway or bench.

Incorrectly-dug swales can cause flooding and severe erosion, so you cannot just dig one that looks like it's probably level. Don't just eyeball it and hope it's on contour. You need to know what you are doing and design swales on contour, or know how to properly design them off contour, to get the results you want. At best, they will just be a waste of your time and effort and will not work to hold moisture in the soil. At worst, they can cause widespread damage and ruin more than your day.

## Gabions

Gabions are cages, cylinders, or other forms filled with rocks or concrete to create a structure used to stop soil erosion. In permaculture landscape, gabions are leaky rock walls that act like semi-permeable dams. They are often placed in valleys or canyons in arid landscapes, in places where water can be dammed.

Because the moisture seeps through the stones slowly, the rest of the water collects behind the obstruction, depositing organic material there. Normally, this organic material would be washed away in a flood, or blown away by desert winds.

Collecting water in this way allows the water to be used over a longer period of time than if it were just allowed to flow down the normal path, unobstructed. Often, plants spring up in the area to take advantage of the moisture, and crabs and shellfish begin to fill the ecosystem.

Species of trees that survive in that climate can be planted along the edges of the gabion, providing food, habitat for animals, nitrogen, and reducing evaporation. Moisture retained in the soil below can continue to keep the trees alive even after the surface water has evaporated.

By capturing naturally-occurring water, you create an oasis in the desert, stopping erosion and further damage and degradation.  Eventually, you reforest the desert, not only preventing desertification, but actually reversing it.

Again, make sure to thoroughly research these principles before attempting any modifications.  If you have a large property, find a way to take a permaculture course or work with a designer or consultant.

# CHAPTER 10

## Planting:  The What, Where, How and Why

What do you include in your garden?  What kinds of plants are best?  Are any varieties better than others in reducing water usage?  Should you use seeds or transplants?  Let's find out.

## What to plant

## Choosing what to grow

It seems pretty obvious, but grow what you like.  If you hate turnips, don't grow them just because they are easy to grow. (And when the seed catalog says, "Even if you don't like turnips, you'll like these"...don't believe it!)

If you grow what you like to eat, drink, smell, or look at, you'll have more enthusiasm for your garden and be more willing to continue when you encounter challenges (which you will).  You can always experiment with new foods and varieties, and I hope you do.  Diversity is important for the planet, and it also boosts your soul.  How exciting it is to grow something new and watch it grow and thrive?  And then you eat it and discover you love it!

If you're the type that does not like new things, I have this advice:  what if this new thing turns out to be the best thing you ever tasted?  You wouldn't experience that if you didn't try it. You'll never know.  Don't let that chance pass you by!

### Look at natives

Plants that are native to your part of the world are already adapted to local conditions.    They have survived with fluctuations of temperature and weather, become adapted to pests and diseases, and already thrive without your help. There may not be many specific vegetables that grow wild, but there will definitely be foods that residents have survived on for generations. Consider growing those first, as you are more likely to be successful with them.

## Consider perennials

Most of what we think of as vegetables are annuals, which need to be planted anew every year. But there are some crops, such as asparagus and rhubarb, which can keep growing and will continue to produce food for many years.

Perennial vegetables are often in the form of spreading ground covers, shrubs, and trees. They can be planted and harvested multiple times in a year. In areas where temperatures are moderate, including tropical parts of the world, perennials can be harvested year-round, providing food with a fraction of the effort of a traditional garden.

Find out what kind of perennial vegetables you can grow in your area. They are often easy to grow, produce abundantly, and are resistant to pest damage, unlike some "normal" vegetables, which can be particular and prone to disease.

Perennials may take some getting used to, because they don't get the media coverage that typical annual vegetables do. (When was the last time you saw a recipe for Okinawan Spinach Soup, or Stir-Fried Katuk?) But they can usually replace other vegetables. In the case of Okinawan spinach, they are a decent substitute for spinach or other leafy greens in recipes.

Consider growing a few perennials along with your normal annual mix. It's nice to have them to fall back on when your gardening efforts fail. If slugs and snails, poor germination, scheduling difficulties, or diseases destroy all your seedlings, leaving you with nothing to plant, you can still eat the perennials you've been ignoring all along.

## Think small and fast

Choose varieties that produce smaller fruit. You will have fewer problems with getting something to harvest, because the fruits will take less time to mature, which means less can go wrong. And smaller plants need less water.

Choose varieties that mature quickly. Some of the fastest-growing crops are leaf lettuce, mizuna, cress, bok choy and some Chinese cabbages, radishes, arugula, some beans, daikon, and turnip greens. Many of these are ready to eat in 50-60 days, and if you start picking young and small, you will have something to munch on after about 30 days.

## Warm climate varieties

Generally speaking, varieties that do better in hotter climates are more tolerant of drought. Varieties that are used to temperate conditions are not.

An old squash variety that has been grown in the desert will be more used to less rainfall than a variety used to growing in cool mountains. But some plants may surprise you. Kale, which likes a bit of frost to sweeten it up, tends to do better in heat and drought than many other greens do.

## How much sunlight?

You'll also need to choose what to grow based on the amount of space you have, how much sun you get, and how long a growing period you have. There is some leeway. You'll still get something to harvest in less-than-ideal conditions, but when conditions are favorable, you will be astounded at how much you can harvest.

This is not an overall how-to-garden book, so you will need to look elsewhere for those guidelines. But here is a list of common garden vegetables and how many hours of full sunlight they need in order to be productive. In general, leaf and root vegetables can tolerate some shade.  Fruiting vegetables (tomatoes, eggplant, peppers) need lots of full sun.

## 4 hours = some sun/some shade is okay:
## Greens
Arugula--welcomes shade; gets bitter in heat

Chives

Cilantro

Collards

Cress

Endive

Green onions/scallions

Kale

Lemon balm

Lettuce

Mint

Mustard greens

Oregano

Parsley

Spinach--welcomes shade; bolts in heat

Swiss chard

## 6 hours = full sun most of the day:
## Root vegetables
Beans

Beets

Broccoli

Brussels sprouts

Carrots

Cauliflower

Daikon

Kohlrabi

Parsnips

Peas

Radishes

Rutabega

Strawberries

Turnips

## 8 hours = full sun all day: Fruiting vegetables

Corn

Cucumbers

Eggplant

Peppers

Pumpkin

Squash

Tomatoes

## Seeds or seedlings?

You can start plants in the garden (or containers) by either planting seeds directly into the ground, or by transplanting seedlings, small plants. Which to use depends on a number of factors.

### Seeds

Seeds are cheaper and easy to obtain. You can often find seeds at a local hardware store, grocery store, department store, or nursery. There are also many mail-order seed companies which provide an even wider selection of seeds than you could ever imagine.

Seeds need to remain moist or mostly moist until they germinate, and germination can be tricky. Some seeds need light to germinate, so you should not cover them with growing medium.

Others need a period of cold in order to germinate, although this is usually only for some shrubs and fruit trees. Other seeds like scarification, which is some scratching up or otherwise penetrating the hard seed coat so that moisture can enter, causing germination.

This can be done by gently scratching with some sandpaper, or carefully cutting off a tiny piece of the seed coat with a sharp utility knife. Most seeds that require light, cool storage, or scarification will say so on the packet instructions.

Because seeds need to remain moist, many people choose to start them in smaller containers or flats (in a tray) and then transplant them into bigger pots, or into the ground, once they are large enough. That is usually when they get their second set of leaves, or five leaves total.

Seeds can also be started indoors, using either natural light, or light fixtures, to get a head start on the weather. In areas where growing seasons are short, starting seeds indoors allows you to start growing before the soil has thawed and is ready to plant.

## Seedlings

Seedlings have already had several weeks of growth behind them when they get transplanted into the ground or a large container. Having transplants ready to go increases productivity in the garden. When something is ready to harvest, gets overrun with disease, is destroyed by pests, or has run its course, by having another plant ready to fill that space in the garden, you do not waste any potential.

Seedlings are also efficient when you do not have enough time to start plants from seed. You can purchase ready-to-plant starters from a home center or nursery and have food almost immediately.

They work well if you have very little space, too. It takes a bit of room and planning to have seeds started and going for everything you want to grow. Buying transplants means you don't need space and resources to start your own seeds.

But many times, purchased seedlings are root-bound in their pots, which reduces their potential growth and productivity. (Root-bound is when you see roots that have been growing around and around in the container, looking for room to expand). So you may choose to grow your own seedlings to get the healthiest starts possible.

## Open-pollinated or heirlooms

Open-pollinated plants are those that are pollinated naturally, by insects such as bees, butterflies, and moths. Heirlooms are open-pollinated varieties that have been passed down through families for generations.

Often these seeds have travelled with family members as they have moved to new areas. The seeds are kept from plants every growing season and used to start plants the following year. In this way, seeds become well adapted to the area in which they are grown, becoming resistant to pests and disease and thriving on local temperatures and humidity.

## Drought-resistant versus drought-tolerant

What's the difference between the two? Drought-tolerant plants are those that can survive in arid places with very little annual rainfall. Typically, these are succulents or other species adapted to a desert environment.

Drought-resistant plants are those that are more likely to survive long periods without water. The plants must be established, however. Few seedlings or newly transplanted plants can survive water shortages.

Both drought-tolerant and drought-resistant plants need to be watered, especially until they are established.  And both will do better with irrigation.   People are quick to plant drought-tolerant plants but do not realize that one of the things many of these plants do to survive is drop their leaves, or go into a state of dormancy, which can leave them looking bare and unhealthy.

In fact, people can unknowingly end up using more water with drought-tolerant plants, trying to get them to look "normal," than they can if they had normal, non-adapted varieties.  At any rate, there are not many vegetable or food crops that are drought-tolerant.  We cover them later in this chapter.

## Drought-resistant or normal?

The whole drought-resistant versus drought-tolerant issue leads to another question.  Should you even bother to choose drought-resistant plants for your garden, or just plant "normal" varieties?

Because healthy, organic garden soil has tremendous water-holding capacity, it should in theory be able to sustain any type of plant, no matter its water demands.  Some gardeners do not change what they plant to accommodate drought, and they claim they have no problems needing to irrigate any more than normally.

On the other hand, it might make sense to choose varieties that have done well for other gardeners in areas with less rainfall.  Often that also means a greater tolerance to heat.  And some of those plants have survived in areas which get periods of high humidity, too, which can lead to more fungal diseases in non-resistant varieties.

So the next section contains a listing of both drought-resistant plants, and specific varieties, where applicable, of those plants.  These have been reported to do well from gardeners around the world.

Of course, since every garden differs, you will need to find out what works for you. What works well in the humid south may do great in southeast Asia, but not so much in Maine. Then again, it might! You won't know until you try. Every gardener has a list of favorite varieties that have come through for them despite the weather, disease, and pests from year to year.

One other tip: if you do choose to plant drought-resistant varieties, be sure to include some "normal" plants too. Weather is highly unpredictable, so although drought may be predicted to continue, a sudden deluge or change in the weather can throw your garden into chaos.

Biodiversity is the key to success, in the world at large, and in your garden. The more different plants and varieties you have growing, the more likely you are to end up with something to harvest, despite whatever Mother Nature throws at you.

## Drought- and heat-tolerant varieties

When you choose varieties for your garden, look for the words "heat-loving," "drought-tolerant," and "sun-loving." Also look for varieties that have done well in similar climates to yours.

Here are some vegetables and specific varieties that other gardeners have reported to have success with. You can try some of them in your garden and see how they do for you.

One thing to keep in mind is invasive species. Some plants do so well that they are considered weeds in parts of the world. They can overtake native vegetation and really screw up the ecosystem. So always heed warnings if a species is considered invasive.

Do an online search for your state's black list, since they differ from area to area. Avoid using plants that are considered invasive weeds. Or if you do grow them, be sure to keep them well contained and managed.

**Plants that tolerate heat and drought well:**

I have not included trees here, but it is important to note that many trees that produce edible crops can be drought tolerant or resistant. If you have the ability to grow trees on your property, look into using permaculture or natural gardening principles to direct and hold rainwater. Those will help any trees you plant, including drought-tolerant ones, such as olive, fig, and date and coconut palms, to survive well.

## Vegetables

Amaranth--can be grown for spinach-like leaves, grain-like seeds, or both

Asparagus

Beans

Corn (old native varieties)

Cowpeas or black-eyed peas

Jalapeno peppers

Long beans (also known as asparagus beans or yard-long beans)

Malabar spinach

Moth beans

Mustard

New Zealand spinach (also known as Warrigal greens, Warrigal cabbage, sea spinach, Cook's cabbage, Botany Bay spinach, *kokihi*, and tetragon)--will grow where there is salt in the soil

Okra (also known as ladies' fingers, bhindi, bamia, or gumbo)

Peppers

Pigeon peas (also known as gandul, guandu, congo bean, red gram)--very drought tolerant, can be cut and used as a mulch to add nitrogen to the soil. The peas provide food and fodder for much of the tropical world.

Pumpkins

Sweet potato

Swiss chard (benefits from a little shade, and stems make an easier-to-grow substitute for celery)

Tepary beans--for dry, sandy soils; they do not like clay soils

Tomatoes

## Flowers

Calendula

California native flowers and plants

California poppy

Desert mallow

Gaillardia

Lantana

Moonflowers (the night-blooming relatives of morning glories)

Morning glories

Osteospermum

Salvias

Sunflowers

Tithonia (also known as Mexican sunflower)

## Herbs

Basil

Lavender

Lemongrass

Parsley

Purslane (also known as verdolaga, pigweed, little hogweed, fatweed, wild portulaca, pussley, or pursley)--a very common, extremely nutritious weed

Rosemary

Sage

Sorrel

Thyme

## Fruits and other

Aloe vera (medicinal, not edible like a vegetable)

Foxtail millet, *Setaria italica* (also known as Italian millet, German millet, Chinese millet, and Hungarian millet)

Litchi tomato

Marigold

Passionfruit

Peanuts (also known as groundnuts)

Pepino (also known as pepino melon and sweet pepino)

Pitaya (also known as pitahaya and dragon fruit)

Pomegranate

Prickly pear (also known as *Opuntia*, paddle cactus, or *nopales*)

Proso millet, *Panicum miliaceum* (also known as common millet, hog millet, and white millet)

Rhubarb

Teff (also known as lovegrass, taf, *mil ethipiene*, and annual bunch grass)

Watermelons (small)

## Specific varieties:

Alabama Blackeyed Bean

Anasazi Sweet Corn

Arkansas Traveler Tomato

Armenian Cucumber

Beit Alpha Cucumber

Christmas Lima Bean

Cocozelle Summer Bush Zucchini

Jimmy Nardello's Sweet Pepper

Kentucky Wonder Pole Bean

Lacinato Kale (also known as Dinosaur Kale)

Lebanese White Bush Marrow Squash

Marconi Peppers
Mexican Sour Gherkin
Perpetual Spinach Chard
Pinky Popcorn
Rattlesnake Pole Bean
Red Russian Kale
Sugar Baby Watermelon
Thai Chili Peppers
Waimanalo Long Eggplant

## Garden buddies: Companion planting for a harmonious garden

Many gardeners swear that certain vegetables, flowers and plants do better or worse when they grow near certain other ones. Since most people seem to take a liking to, or dislike, certain other people, why shouldn't plants also have their favorites?

Some plants help by attracting beneficial insects or repelling harmful ones. Marigolds remove harmful nematodes from the soil, but they need to be planted where nematode damage has been found, and they need a full season to have the best effect.

There is still so much we do not know about the natural world, and we have only a glimpse of how companion planting works. But here are some companion planting suggestions to try in your garden.

### Asparagus

*Likes:* tomatoes, parsley, and basil.

## Beans

*Likes:* carrots, beets, and cauliflower. They benefit from marigolds and summer savory.

*Do not like:* gladiolas and any member of the onion family, including garlic, leeks, chives.

## Bush beans

*Likes:* do well when planted with cucumbers and strawberries.

*Do not like:* fennel.

## Pole beans

*Do not like:* sunflowers or kohlrabi.

## Beets

*Likes:* bush beans, onions, and kohlrabi.

*Do not like:* pole beans.

## Cabbage

*Likes:* beans, potatoes, herbs, especially sage.

## Cabbage family plants, including cauliflower, broccoli, kale, kohlrabi, collards, Brussels sprouts, turnips, rutabegas

*Likes:* hyssop, thyme, wormwood to repel white cabbage butterflies, whose caterpillars can destroy a crop. They also like aromatic plants or those with many blossoms, including dill, sage, peppermint, and rosemary.

*Do not like:* strawberries, tomatoes, pole beans.

# Carrots

*Likes:* onions, leeks, sage, rosemary, wormwood to repel carrot flies, leaf lettuce, chives, radishes, peas

*Do not like:* dill

# Cauliflower

*Likes:* celery

*Does not like:* tomatoes, strawberries

# Collards

*Likes:* interplanting with tomatoes

# Sweet corn

*Likes:* potatoes, peas, beans, cucumbers, pumpkin, squash, sunflowers

*Does not like:* tomatoes

# Cucumbers

*Likes:* beans, peas, chives, cabbage, potatoes

# Garlic

*Does not like:* beans and peas

# Lettuce

*Likes:* carrots and radishes

## Onions

*Likes:* carrots

## Peas

*Likes:* carrots, sweet corn, turnips, beans, cucumbers

*Do not like:* onions, shallots, garlic

## Potatoes

*Likes:* beans, peas, sweet corn, cabbage

*Do not like:* tomatoes, sunflowers

## Pumpkin

*Likes:* sweet corn

## Tomatoes

*Likes:* basil, asparagus, carrots, parsley

*Do not like:* kohlrabi, potatoes

## The three sisters

Native American Indians have used a companion planting system including what they call the "three sisters"--corn, which is sometimes substituted by sunflowers, beans, and pumpkin or squash.

The corn or sunflowers provide something for the beans to climb on. The beans affix nitrogen to the soil. The large leaves of the pumpkin or squash act as a living mulch to shade the ground, retaining moisture and reducing weeds.

Also, all three of these could be eaten fresh, or dried or stored, for long-term food. They were planted just before the annual rains, which provided moisture in an otherwise arid climate.

## Beneficial attractors

Be sure to add some plants that will attract beneficial insects, including pollinators, to your garden. Bees are the most well-known pollinators, but moths, butterflies, and other insects also help.

Without adequate pollinators, you will not be able to get any fruits. By that, I refer to the biological definition of fruits--the fleshy, seed-containing part of a flowering plant.

So it does include what we normally consider to be "fruits"--grapes, strawberries, figs, peaches, and plums. But it also means "fruits" that we normally consider to be "vegetables"--eggplant, peppers, cucumbers, tomatoes, beans, peas. Plus other herbs, nuts, flowers, and grains--sunflowers, walnuts, corn, wheat, dill--and things we don't eat, such as cotton.

Without pollinators, we'd have a tough time surviving. So you want to do what you can to encourage them.

Be sure to add flowers such as marigolds, alyssum, cosmos, and sunflowers. Many herbs are attractants too, and the added benefit is that you can eat them, use them in teas, throw their flowers in salads, or use them medicinally. Pollinator-attracting herbs include dill, borage, anise hyssop, fennel, and Italian parsley.

Other beneficial insects will also be drawn to your garden. Some of them prey on harmful pest species, so planting attractors has multiple benefits.

## Tips for healthy seedlings

***Provide lots of light.*** Seedlings that do not have enough light grow leggy. They get tall and thin and do not do well when they are moved to the bright outside sunlight.

***Keep moist.*** Seedlings are so tiny and weak that they can dry out and die if you miss just one day, or even several hours, of watering.

***Do not overwater.*** Especially if you start seeds indoors, you can kill seeds by too much watering. Excess moisture also encourages dampening off, a fungal disease that kills seedlings.

***Thin to the strongest two or three*** if you have planted more seeds than that in one container or area. Otherwise, they compete for space and growth and none of them develop well. When transplanting, use only the healthiest one, or separate them, being careful not to destroy their roots.

***Water seedlings well*** after transplanting them. This reduces the shock of moving and helps them get established in a new area.

## Where to plant

Put plants that have the same moisture and warmth requirements together in the same area. That helps to create microclimates. For example, eggplants, peppers, and tomatoes prefer warm days and cool nights, and require moderate watering.

Place seedlings that will become larger plants at the rear of your sections or containers, so that as they grow, they will not shade out other plants. On the other hand, if you want them to provide some shade to your plants as they grow, you'd want them in front.

The south-facing side of any area will get more sunlight, and the north will get the least. For that reason, orient your gardens to face south, and place pathways running east to west, whenever possible.

## When to plant

The best time to plant, whether seeds or seedlings, is just before it rains. If you have an annual rainy season, plant to coincide with that.

The ancient Hopi Indians of Arizona planted two crops a year, to coincide with annual spring and summer rains. They also knew that their soil had the capacity to hold onto moisture, and by understanding how this worked, they could us a method of dry farming that produced food in a desert area.

Other than before a rain, it's better to plant in the cooler seasons of the year in your area, especially if you live where summer temperatures soar. Plant early in the season, so that plant roots will get a chance to go deep, and plants can become established before it gets hot.

In northern climates, plant as early as possible for your area. Gardeners in more northern zones often have a shorter overall growing season but do not get as high temperatures as some areas in the south.

Most people grow in the spring through the summer months. But don't feel you need to follow the norm if it doesn't work well in your area. Avoiding the summer heat, and planting in the fall or winter works well for many gardeners who live in the southern part of the U.S., the tropics, or areas of southeast Asia where temperatures tend to be warm to hot, with high humidity, most of the year. Taking advantage of cooler weather during winter months makes for an easier harvest, using less water.

Plant early in the morning or later in the afternoon, so that seeds and transplants won't get burned up by the heat. Be sure to drench the area well, so they have lots of water to soak up.

## How to plant

Make a hole large and deep enough to accommodate the new transplant. If you're using newspaper pots, plant the whole thing, or carefully tear off any of the pot that is not enmeshed with roots.

Tap the sides of a plastic pot with the side of a trowel. Turn the pot upside-down and carefully remove the plant.

Place plants in the ground so that they are the same depth in the new soil as they were in the old soil. Press the soil down around them firmly but not too much. You want them to stay in place, but you do not want to compact the soil.

Give them a good soaking, to help them get established in their new home. Singing them a song and expressing your gratitude probably won't hurt, either, although you might want to be sure none of your neighbors are watching you, before you do!

## Tips for pepper and tomato seedlings

Tomatoes and peppers will start to produce roots on their stems wherever they touch the ground. You can use this to your advantage when starting seeds in order to produce a seedling that is loaded with roots by the time you transplant it into the garden. This means the plant will be able to support tremendous life as it grows, producing a more bountiful harvest.

Rather than filling an entire pot, start your seeds in just a small amount of growing medium. As the seedling gets taller, fill in around the stem with more soil. This will encourage more root growth. Continue to do this in stages, until you have filled the pot. When you transplant the seedling, bury the entire thing, up to the bottom-most leaves, in the soil.

## Air pruning

When roots are grown in containers, they can become root-bound. This is when roots hit the side of the container and end up growing around in circles, in a futile effort to find more nutrients in order to support the plant.

If you've ever bought small transplants from a garden store, or larger potted plants, you've seen the tangle of matted roots when you pulled the seedling out of the pot. Some plants even stop growing when they hit this barrier, and they end up stunted.

Air pruning happens when roots hit air pockets in the soil. The root tips die off, but sprout more side roots further back. When this happens repeatedly, a plant ends up with a bountiful, dense root system that increases production and produces a heartier plant.

Commercial nurseries have used this principle to their advantage with tree seedlings. By encouraging air pruning, they can make the largest tree in the shortest amount of time, which means they can charge you more for them.

You can encourage air pruning in your plants by creating more exposure to air. There are commercial pot systems that look like plastic pots covered with tunnel-like holes.

Some gardeners have experimented with drilling multiple tiny holes in the sides of plastic pots, then using a liner of weed-barrier fabric inside to keep the growing medium from falling through the holes. The same effect can be obtained by growing in woven bags. You might want to experiment with either of these methods.

# CHAPTER 11

## General Gardening Tips

Although this is not a general gardening book, here are a few helpful tips that can make your growing easier and more productive.

### Pest control

***Grow a variety of plants.*** Doing so will increase the odds that whatever pest species you end up with will also be countered by a beneficial species to keep it in check. It also means if you have a crop failure, there will be something else that survives and allows you to have a harvest.

***Grow beneficial attractants,*** such as flowering plants and lots of herbs. Some herbs actually repel the "bad" bugs.

***Become a pest detective.*** Go out and watch what's happening on, around, and under your plants at different times during the day. Go out at night, too. Pests are easier to control when caught early, before they become too plentiful.

***Use hand picking*** and destroying whenever possible. It's very easy to go out at night with a knife and flashlight and slice through slugs. It costs you nothing but time and effort, and it's highly effective.

***Healthy soil begets healthy plants.*** Healthy plants do not fall prey to diseases and insects as much as weak plants do. And healthy soil begets healthy plants.

# Gardening on a budget

## Reuse materials whenever possible

All organic materials that pass your way can be put into the garden. Use kitchen scraps, weeds, wilted leaves, coffee grounds, shredded paper, shredded newspaper, egg shells, and pistachio nut shells. (Can you tell what I've been snacking on lately)?!

Inorganic materials, such as plastic, can also be reused. But you need to decide if the risk of chemicals leaching from the plastics is worth taking if you use them to hold water or as containers to garden in.

## Be careful of free stuff

Be wary of picking up bags of leaves, grass clippings, free manure, or compost, unless you are absolutely sure they do not contain any pesticides, herbicides, fungicides, growth enhancers, or other synthetic chemicals. Powerful chemicals created by the big companies stay in the soil for years, killing microbial life.

Some gardeners in New Zealand, Great Britain, and parts of the U.S., including Vermont, Montana, Pennsylvania, North Carolina, California, and Washington, have ruined their garden soil by adding free material that killed all their plants and destroyed soil fertility. The problem has also been traced to tainted manure in commercial compost.

When potent herbicides are sprayed onto hayfields and pastures and cows eat them, the chemical remains poisonous for years. Even after the cow manure has been composted, it continues to kill seedlings.

The active ingredients to watch out for are picloram, clopyralid, and aminopyralid. If you get any hay, compost, or manure, be sure to check with your sources to see if any of these active ingredients were used. If so, let them know how dangerous these chemicals are, and stay away from their products.

You might want to grow a separate test section with free materials, just to be sure there are no problems. Plant bean or pea seeds in some containers, using the free materials as part of your growing mix. Plant other identical containers, using your own safe growing medium. Label which is which.

Seed germination will be poor, and plant leaves will curl if there is contamination. Some plants, such as tomatoes, beans, peas, eggplant, sunflowers, potatoes, and peppers, are more affected than others.

If you do see damage, throw everything out and stay away from that source in the future. You can also file an incident report with the Environmental Protection Agency. You can find the link at the back of this book.

## Reuse discarded toilet tanks

(and bowls, if you are not too queasy to do so) as planters. They have a large capacity, get thrown out all over the place, are glazed, so they hold water well, and are free.

If you just want the tanks (which also stack nicely together side by side), you will need to separate them from the bowls, or just use those that are already detached. Take out the hardware from inside, and add a piece of weed-barrier fabric underneath, to prevent weeds from coming up.

Add something in the bottom hole to prevent all your soil from draining away. Another piece of weed-barrier fabric, or some reused old window screen works well.

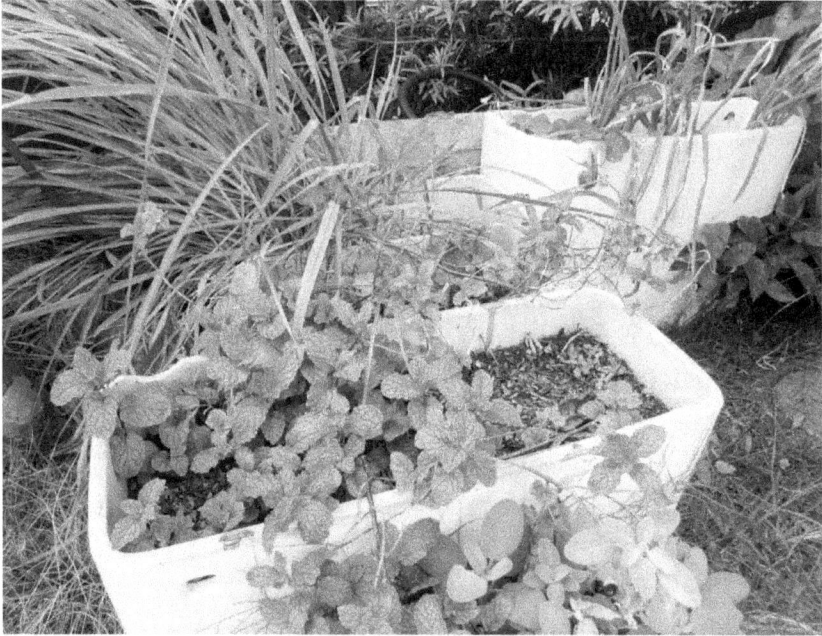

Reusing toilet tanks as free planters for drought-resistant herbs. Back right: green onions. Left, back to front: lemongrass, spearmint, sage.

## Free seeds

You can, of course, save your own seeds. Some of the easiest to save are lettuce, dill, fennel, basil, escarole, calendula, coriander, pumpkins, squash, cucumbers, melons, beans, peppers, and tomatoes.

Every time you save seeds from your own plants, you increase the ability of the next generation to adapt to your local conditions. Over time, you get plants that like your soil's natural composition, local weather and temperature variations.

You can also trade seeds with other gardeners in your area or from other parts of the world. Many people, especially urban gardeners, do not need all the seeds in one packet. By using some and trading the rest, you can increase your supply, for reduced cost.

## Keep seeds dry and cool

We keep our seeds in the refrigerator, because the high outside humidity in the tropics shortens the lifespan of our seeds. You may just want to put them into a sealed glass or plastic container and in a cool part of the house.

## Find sources for more organic materials

Is there a raw-foods or organic restaurant nearby? Ask if they have extra throwaways and scraps that you can have. How about a coffee shop? What do they do with their coffee grounds?

Check with your city or county extension service or zoo. Is there a place you can get wood chips, compost, or composted animal manure? Sometimes it's free for the taking.

## Start new plants from old

Use what you buy at the store to start new plants. Lemongrass, basil, and mint can all be started by putting a stem into a glass of water until roots form. Change the water daily to prevent rotting, then transplant to your garden once roots form. The bottoms of green onions (with roots) can be planted in a pot of growing medium.

## What to do with your harvest

Just in case your gardening efforts have you overloaded with zucchini, or something similar, that you don't know what to do with, here are a few ideas for excess harvest.

## Food preservation methods

You can freeze, pickle, can, lactic-acid ferment, or dry excess produce. You can make wine, juice, herbal teas, vinegar, ice cream, breads, soups. Throw purees into everything you make. Tomato, spinach, pumpkin, zucchini, apple, carrot, and pear purees work great in brownies, muffins, and cakes.

See my book, ***The New Scoop: Recipes for Dairy-Free, Vegan Ice Cream in Unusual Flavors (Plus Some Old Favorites)***, for ice cream, sherbet, sorbet, and frozen yogurt recipes using fruits, vegetables, and herbs. Favorites include Cucumber-Mint Frozen Yogurt, Sweet Potato Ice Cream, and Strawberry Basil Balsamic Ice Cream.

## Donate

Give some to neighbors, friends, family, or a shelter that feeds the homeless. Bring a bucket full to the office, social dance, church, birthday party, or meeting.

## Sell

Ask a local restaurant or store if they want to buy your produce. Wholesale prices are usually one-third to one-half of retail. Fresh herbs are always in demand at fancier restaurants.

# CHAPTER 12

## Learn More:  Resources

The best way to find out what to grow, learn about new varieties to try, or glean helpful tips and tricks, is to network with other gardeners. Even if you do not learn something new, you may be inspired by other people's successes or failures.

### In person

### Take a walk

The best way to meet others with information that can help you is to find other gardeners in your area. Keep your eyes open as you drive anywhere.  Even better, take walks around your neighborhood and other nearby areas.  The slow pace of walking allows you to notice plants and gardens that you cannot see (or smell) from your vehicle.

You can discover all sorts of plants that are doing well in your area, which means there is the potential for you to grow them, too. If you're lucky, you may even get to speak to the gardener and talk shop.  Ask them about any special needs the plant has, find out what it's called, how to cook it, etc.

In our area, there are a lot of immigrant families from Asia and other Pacific Islands.  I've learned about all kinds of different Filipino, Okinawan, and Chinese vegetables and herbs just from other people who grow them.

### Community gardens

Your community may have garden areas, where people who do not have space to garden at home can have a plot of their own to tend. Take a stroll through your local gardens and see what people are growing, how they stake their vegetables up, and stop to smell the roses, lavender, or other fragrant herbs and flowers when you see them.

If you are there during early morning or early evening, you are more likely to see people working in their gardens and can ask them questions or strike up a conversation. I've also had people offer to share seeds or cuttings with me, so that I can try to grow them in my own space.

## Board of Water Supply

Our local Board of Water Supply has a demonstration xeriscape garden, where they do occasional tours and classes. There we can see examples of plants that grow easily in our area that need little to no additional watering. While these plants usually are not for eating, it may be informative and helpful in other ways. You might, for example, find out some tips and tricks for conserving water.

## Local nurseries and garden centers

In addition to being a source for plants to purchase, a local grow center may have someone knowledgeable you can talk with. Sometimes a worker is available to speak to. You may run into a grower, coming to refill the shelves, or find another customer browsing. All of these people may be able to give you tidbits of helpful information, if you are brave enough to ask.

## University Extension Offices

Most universities have an extension office or college or department of agriculture. They are a great source of information specific to your area. Often they sell seeds or plants which have been developed or bred to do well in your part of the world.

Sometimes they may offer classes which you can take free, not for university credits.  Or they may offer online learning, classes which are broadcast by your local television or cable station.

This is also the best place to go for identifying local insect pests, unknown plant species, or diseases.  Sometimes you need to jump through hoops to find contact information, but these are the most academic, educated sources in your area, if you can ever figure out how to reach them!

They are also a source for online information, usually in the form of downloadable pdf files.  Contact your local university, or do a search for "extension office" and your state.

## Online

## Gardening forums

There is a ton of useful information out there, and there are many people who visit forums daily or regularly, sharing their knowledge and expertise.  It's also a way to connect with others in your area that you might otherwise never even know existed.

It's so easy to get lost and spend more time than you intended, since others will post a thread about something called "hugelculture," for example, which you may never have heard of before.  So you click the link and then disappear for the next three days, learning all you can about this new, shiny object!

Here are some of the most active, helpful garden forums:

### I Dig My Garden

http://idigmygarden.com/forums/

This is the forum connected to Baker Creek Heirloom Seeds. There are many members all over the U.S. as well as internationally, and most of them are interested in growing rare and unusual varieties. Stay away from the recipe section. Don't say I didn't warn you!

### Dave's Garden

http://davesgarden.com/community/forums/

Here you can find 216 different forums, including some on specific types of plants, such as fruits and nuts, or legumes.

### Garden Web

http://forums.gardenweb.com/forums/

An extensive selection of topics.

### Kitchen Gardens International

http://kgi.org

Sort of a forum mixed together with links, blog posts, and other information.

### Permies

http://www.permies.com/

Permaculture and beyond-the-garden information, such as building, alternative energy, and homesteading.


## Sources for Seeds

Here are some of my favorite sources for vegetable and herb seeds.

### Baker Creek Heirloom Seeds

http://www.rareseeds.com/
Phone: (417) 924-8917

All of their seeds are non-hybrid and non-GMOs. They have an extensive selection, a stunning catalog, and multiple international varieties, many of which are rare and hard to find.

## Ecology Action

http://www.bountifulgardens.org/

Phone: (707) 459-6410

Heirloom and open-pollinated seeds. They have the best offering of cover crops and grains.

## Johnny's Selected Seeds

http://www.johnnyseeds.com/

Phone: (877) 564-6697

Non-GMO seeds, although some are hybrids. They are in Maine, so this is a good company if you live in northern climates.

## Native Seeds/SEARCH

https://www.nativeseeds.org

Phone: (520) 622-0830

They specialize in non-GMO, open-pollinated and heirloom seeds of the general Southwest. If you are looking for tepary beans, they sell them here, plus many Mexican varieties of vegetables and herbs, corn, and popcorn!

## Nichol's Garden Nursery

https://www.nicholsgardennursery.com/store/index.php

Phone: (800) 422-3985

They specialize in herb seeds and plants, but they also sell a great variety of other things, including kits for beer, cheese, and winemaking.

## Pinetree Garden Seeds

http://www.superseeds.com/

Phone: (207) 926-3400

Non-GMO seeds, although some are hybrids. They have lower prices and fewer seeds in each packet than most of the other companies, which is helpful if you want to try new things.

## Seed Savers Exchange

http://www.seedsavers.org/

Phone: (563) 382-5990

Members of this organization are committed to saving seeds from heirloom and often endangered varieties. You can shop their catalog without being a member.

## Southern Exposure Seed Exchange

http://www.southernexposure.com

Phone: (540) 894-9480

Selling non-GMO seeds, almost all are open-pollinated or heirloom, adapted to the southeastern U.S. and mid-Atlantic regions.

# Links to more information online

Disclaimer: Some of these links are affiliate links. That means if you click on one and buy something, I may get a small commission. Thank you for your support.

## USDA code of federal regulations for organic products:

http://tinyurl.com/kvr484u

## Food recalls:

http://www.foodsafety.gov/recalls/recent/

http://www.fsis.usda.gov/wps/portal/fsis/topics/recall
s-and-public-health-alerts/current-recalls-and-alerts

## Information on the Al Baydha project:

http://www.permacultureglobal.com/projects/286-al-
baydha-project

http://www.youtube.com/user/albaydha

## Bacteria:

http://ed.ted.com/lessons/how-bacteria-talk-bonnie-
bassler

A fascinating talk on bacterial communication that has very
little to do with gardening but very much to do with you and
your body

## Bottle tower gardens:

http://containergardening.wordpress.com/2011/09/07/
bottle-tower-gardening-how-to-start-willem-van-cotthem/

http://edis.ifas.ufl.edu/hs1186

## Keyhole gardens:

http://www.debtolman.com/FieldGuide.pdf

http://www.sendacow.org.uk/lessonsfromafrica/resour
ces/keyhole-gardens

## Spiral gardens:

http://frugalkiwi.co.nz/2012/01/building-a-herb-spiral/
http://ecologiadesign.com/2013/04/20/herb-spirals/

**A 5-gallon bucket with drip irrigation:**

https://www.csupomona.edu/~jskoga/dripirrigation/

**Rain barrels:**

http://www.lakesuperiorstreams.org/stormwater/toolk it/rainbarrels.html

**Excellent how-to video for reusing 55-gallon plastic drums:**

https://www.youtube.com/watch?v=vwZ7xr9EUDc

**Drip irrigation using a plastic bag for water:**

http://eosinternational.org/wp-content/uploads/2011/11/EOS-DI-Manual-English.pdf

**Woodchips:**

http://puyallup.wsu.edu/~Linda%20Chalker-Scott/Horticultural%20Myths_files/Myths/magazine%20pdfs/Woodchips.pdf
http://chipdrop.in
Sign up online to have a load of woodchips delivered to you.

**Back to Eden:**

The film about Paul Gautschi, who uses wood chips in his now-famous garden:
http://tinyurl.com/edenfilm

**Fog collectors:**

https://www.youtube.com/watch?v=_Xn7YTzPydE

A video of a fog collection system in Eritrea. It's difficult to understand the narrator's strongly accented English, but there are some good close-up shots where you can see how the system is built.

https://www.youtube.com/watch?v=b8TBdrzemiM

A system set up in the mountains, which irrigates crops downhill.

https://www.youtube.com/watch?v=sdyyw9fe3KI

Fog catchers in the Atacama Desert, the driest desert in the world.

## Gardening myths debunked:

http://puyallup.wsu.edu/~Linda%20Chalker-Scott/Horticultural%20Myths_files/index.html

## Newspaper pot directions for woodturners:

http://hants-woodturners-hwa.co.uk/try-yourself/paper-seed-pot-maker-alan-sturgess/

http://www.highlandwoodworking.com/woodturning-tips-1302feb/curtis.html

http://www.ptwoodturners.org/Tips%20and%20Handouts/Turn%20a%20Pot.pdf

## Make a newspaper pot form using PVC:

http://tendcollective.blogspot.com/2013/04/diy-pvc-paper-pot-maker.html

**Using a can:**

http://www.motherearthnews.com/organic-gardening/easy-newspaper-pots.aspx

**Using a wine bottle:**

http://www.imperfecthomemaking.com/2013/03/news paper-seed-starting-pots.html

**Gabions:**

http://permaculturenews.org/2014/02/15/reversing-desertification-gabions/

**Root development in various crops:**

http://www.soilandhealth.org/01aglibrary/010137veg.r oots/010137toc.html

**Invasive plants lists:**

http://www.fs.fed.us/database/feis/plants/weed/

http://www.invasivespeciesinfo.gov/plants/main.shtml

**Diseases transmitted by mosquitoes:**

http://npic.orst.edu/pest/mosquito/diseases.html

**Sub-irrigation rain gutter system:**

http://www.insideurbangreen.org/2012/04/a-farmer-makes-a-rain-gutter-sub-irrigation-planter-sip-garden-.html

**Commercial sub-irrigated planter kits:**

http://tinyurl.com/sipkits

**Sub-irrigation planter using organic materials:**

https://www.youtube.com/watch?v=wGF72sOwgJI

## Sub-irrigation/air pruning hybrid container:

https://www.youtube.com/watch?v=VPxj8e2r7H0

## Sub-irrigated planters using 5-gallon buckets:

http://www.globalbuckets.org/

## Commercial compost tumblers:

http://tinyurl.com/klq9oka

## Commercial countertop compost systems:

http://tinyurl.com/ljjep3t

## Permaculture video:

Seeds of Permaculture--Tropical Permaculture
https://www.youtube.com/watch?v=2cr10nOm0xU

## Killer compost:

http://tinyurl.com/mw96roa

## File a report if you have been affected by contaminated compost:

http://tinyurl.com/killercompost

# Books

See the Bibliography, which follows, to find books and other publications for in-depth information on any of the topics covered.

# Bibliography

*The Basic Book of Organic Gardening.* Robert Rodale, Editor. Ballantine Books, 1971.

*The Best Place for Garbage: The Essential Guide to Recycling With Composting Worms.* Sandra Wiese. WiR Press, 2011.

*Carrots Love Tomatoes: Secrets of Companion Planting for Successful Gardening.* Louise Riotte. Storey Publishing, LLC, 1998.

*Compost Toilets.* Paul Calvert. Practical Action: The Schumacher Centre for Technology and Development, pdf.

*Construction Manual: Drip Irrigation.* Emerging Opportunities for Sustainability International, pdf.

*Container Vegetable Gardening.* Karen Demboski, Annette Swanberg, Jane C. Martin. Ohio State University Extension, Horticulture and Crop Science Fact Sheet, http://ohioline.osu.edu/hyg-fact/1000/1647.html.

*Drought Tolerant Vegetables.* Ellen Brown. http://www.sustainable-media.com/, pdf.

*Dry-Farming: A System of Agriculture for Countries Under a Low Rainfall.* John Andreas Widtsoe. The Macmillan Company, 1920.

*Esther Deans' Gardening Book: Growing Without Digging.* Esther Dean. Angus and Robertson, 1977.

*Field Guide to How to Build a Keyhole Garden DVD with Debbie Tolman, Ph.D.* Debbie Tolman, pdf.

*A Garden in a Sack: Experiences in Kibera, Nairobi.* Peggy Pascal and Eunice Mwende. Solidarites, pdf.

*How to Build a Keyhole Garden.* Send a Cow, pdf.

*Irrigating (Watering) Your Vegetable Garden.* Heidi Kratsch. University of Nevada Cooperative Extension Fact Sheet-10-16.

*Lasagna Gardening: A New Layering System for Bountiful Gardens: No Digging, No Tilling, No Weeding, No Kidding!* Patricia Lanza. Rodale Books, 1998.

*Mycorrhizae: So, What the Heck Are They, Anyway?* Linda Chalker-Scott. Washington State University, Puyallup Research and Extension Center, pdf.

*The Myth of Permanent Peatlands: "Peat Moss Is An Environmentally Friendly Organic Amendment Essential For Many Horticultural Purposes."* Linda Chalker-Scott. Washington State University, Puyallup Research and Extension Center, pdf.

*The One-Straw Revolution: An Introduction to Natural Farming.* Masanobu Fukuoka. Other India Press, 1992.

*The Organic Gardener's Handbook of Natural Pest and Disease Control: A Complete Guide to Maintaining a Healthy Garden and Yard the Earth-Friendly Way.* Fern Marshall Bradley, Barbara W. Ellis, and Deborah L. Martin. Rodale Books, 2010.

*Perennial Vegetables: From Artichoke to 'Zuika' Taro, a Gardener's Guide to Over 100 Delicious, Easy-to-Grow Edibles.* Eric Toensmeier. Chelsea Green Publishing, 2007.

*Permaculture: A Designers' Manual.* Bill Mollison. Tagari Publications, 1988.

*Plants to Grow in a Keyhole Garden.* Lessons From Africa. Send a Cow, pdf.

*The Principles of Irrigation Practice.* John Andreas Widtsoe. The Macmillan Company, 1914.

*Rainwater Harvesting for Drylands and Beyond (Vol. 2): Water-Harvesting Earthworks.* Brad Lancaster. Rainsource Press, 2007.

*Rodale's Illustrated Encyclopedia of Herbs.* Claire Kowalkchik, William H. Hylton, Anna Carr, Rodale Press. Rodale Press, 2000.

*Saving Water in Vegetable Gardens.* University of California, Vegetable Research Information Center, Department of Vegetable Crops, pdf.

*Soaring Food Prices and Nutrition in Urban Areas: Sack Gardens in Kenya.* FAO Nutrition and Consumer Protection Division (AGN), pdf.

*Solutions for Small Farmers and Home Gardens: Building a Low-Cost Vertical Soilless System for Production of Small Vegetable and Fruit Crops.* Bielinski M. Santos, Teresa P. Salame-Donoso, and Shawn C. Arango. University of Florida IFAS Extension, pdf.

*South Africans Turn to Fog Harvesting for Water.* www.fogharvesting.com, pdf.

*Southern Herb Growing.* Madalene Hill, Gwen Barclay, and Jean Hardy. Shearer Publishing, 1989.

*Square Foot Gardening.* Mel Bartholomew. Cool Springs Press, 2013.

*Using Surface Tension Measurements To Understand How Pollution Can Influence Cloud Formation, Fog, and Precipitation.* Sarah D. Brooks, Marissa Gonzales, and Roberto Farias. Department of Atmospheric Science, Texas A&M University, pdf.

*The Vegetable Gardener's Guide to Permaculture: Creating an Edible Ecosystem.* Christopher Shein and Julie Thompson. Timber Press, 2013.

*Water Conservation in the Vegetable Garden.* Colorado State University Extension, CMG GardenNotes #716.

*Water-Efficient Gardening.* John Marder. The Crowood Press Ltd., 2009.

*Water Harvesting Traditions in the Desert Southwest.* Joel Glanzberg, pdf.

*Wood Chip Mulch: Landscape Boon or Bane?* Linda Chalker-Scott. Washington State University, Puyallup Research and Extension Center. From *MasterGardener,* Summer 2007, pdf.

*Worms Eat My Garbage: How to Set Up and Maintain a Worm Composting System, 2nd Edition.* Mary Appelhof and Mary Frances Fenton. Flower Press, 2003.

# Index

Abraha Aspaha, 32
adaptation, 26
A-frame tool, 108
    calibrating, 109
    using, 110
Africa, 146
    keyhole garden, 97
    sack gardens, 93
agriculture college, 141
Agriculture,U. S. Department of, 16
air conditioners
    reusing water from, 64
air pruning, 92, 133, 150
air    pruning/sub-irrigation
    hybrids, 92
air,importance to plants, 40
Al Baydha, 31, 146
Alabama Blackeyed Bean, 124
alfalfa, 87
algae, 42
    and fog collectors, 68
allergies
    and vegan ice cream, 1
aloe vera, 124
alternative energy, 143
alyssum, 129
amaranth
    and drought resistance, 122
Anasazi Sweet Corn, 124
anise hyssop, 129
annual bunch grass, 124
apple
    in muffins and cakes, 138
aquaponics, 95
Arkansas Traveler Tomato, 124
Armenian Cucumber, 124
arugula, 115
    how much light, 116
    in spiral garden, 101
asparagus, 114

and drought resistance, 122
    companion planting, 125, 128
asparagus beans, 122
asphalt and water runoff, 59
Atacama Desert, 67
Atlantic, mid-, 145
**attracting    beneficial    insects**, 129
azaleas, 50
Back to Eden, 54, 147
backyard gardening, 24
bacteria, 41, 42, 146
    in graywater systems, 64
bags, grow, 91
Baker Creek Heirloom Seeds, 142, 143
baking, 138
baking with fruits and vegetables, 138
bamia, 122
bananas, 26
barrels for rainwater collecting, 65
basil
    companion planting, 125
    drought resistance, 123
    in spiral garden, 101
    starting another plant, 138
Bassler, Bonnie, 41
beans, 115
    Alabama Blackeyed, 124
    and drought resistance, 122
    and the three sisters, 128
    Christmas lima, 124
    companion planting, 126
    how much light, 116
    in hugelkultur, 104
    Kentucky Wonder Pole, 124
    pole, and companion planting, 126
    Rattlesnake Pole, 125

tepary, 144
beans, bush
    companion planting, 126
beer
    bottles, in keyhole garden, 98
beermaking kits, 144
bees, 5, 104, 119, 129
beetles, 25
beets, 50
    companion planting, 126
    how much light, 116
    in square foot garden, 84
Beit Alpha Cucumber, 124
bench in swales, 111
**beneficial insects**, 129
berms, 31
beverage bottles, 146
    in tower garden, 95
    self watering, 89
bhindi, 122
Bill Mollison, 37
biodiversity, 27, 121
birds
    and seed germination, 27
Bisphenol A
    in bottle tower garden, 96
Black Gold, 43
black-eyed peas
    and drought resistance, 122
blueberries, 50
Board of Water Supply, 141
bok choy, 115
bones in keyhole garden, 98
Bonnie Bassler, 41
books in keyhole garden, 98
borage, 129
Botany Bay spinach, 122
bottle, 146
    wine, to make newspaper pots, 149
bottle tower garden, 95
    how to make, 96
bottles

and sub-irrigated planters, 86
    for drip irrigation, 73
    in sub-irrigated planters, 88
    in tower garden, 95
    plastic, self watering, 89
    sub-irrigated, 89
BPA
    in bottle tower garden, 96
branches
    in hugelkultur, 103
    in spiral garden, 100
breads, 138
breaking up the soil with vegetables, 51
bricks
    in keyhole garden, 98
    in spiral garden, 100
broccoli, 50
    companion planting, 126
    contaminated salad kit, 17
    how much light, 116
broken pots, 88
    in spiral garden, 100
brushing your teeth, 62
Brussels sprouts, 50
    companion planting, 126
    how much light, 116
bucket, 147
buckets
    5-gallon sub-irrigated planters, 150
    and sub-irrigated planters, 86
bugs, 134
    bees, 5, 104, 119
    carrot flies, 127
    **pollinators**, 129
    white cabbage butterfly, 126
burdock, 51
bush
    as shade, 57
    to reduce wind, 58
bush beans
    companion planting, 126

bushes to slow water, 60
**butterflies**, 129
cabbage
  Chinese, 115
  companion planting, 126, 127, 128
  in square foot garden, 84
cabbage butterflies, 126
cabbage family
  companion planting, 126
cactus, 26, 52
  and compost, 44
  Opuntia, drought resistance, 124
  paddle, 124
  prickly pear, drought resistance, 124
cakes, 138
calendula, 123
  in spiral garden, 100
calibrating the A-frame tool, 109
California
  radiation from tuna from Japan, 11
California native flowers and plants, 123
California poppy, 123
can
  making newspaper pots from, 149
cans in keyhole garden, 98
carbon materials in compost, 44
cardboard
  and worms, 48
  for sheet mulching, 55
  in keyhole garden, 98
  in lasagna garden, 85
carrot flies, 127
carrots, 51, 59
  companion planting, 126
  how much light, 116
  in muffins and cakes, 138
  in square foot garden, 84

castings, worm, 48
catchers, fog, 67
caterpillars, 126
cauliflower, 50
  companion planting, 126
  how much light, 116
celery
  companion planting, 127
cement
  in keyhole garden, 98
chain, rain, 66
chamomile
  in spiral garden, 101
cheesemaking kits, 144
chicken manure, 48
  in hugelkultur, 103
chickens, 47, 54
  and compost, 45
  and erosion, 61
children, 22
Chile, 67
chili peppers
  jalapenos, 122
  Thai, 125
China, 29
Chinese cabbages, 115
Chinese millet, 124
chips, wood. See wood chips
chives
  companion planting, 126, 127
  how much light, 116
  in sack garden, 94
  in spiral garden, 101
chlorine
  to clean fog collectors, 68
choosing what to grow, 113
Christmas Lima Bean, 124
cilantro
  how much light, 116
  in spiral garden, 101
classes, 141
clay soil, 39
cloth, shade, for shade cover, 57

coconuts, 26, 122
Cocozelle Summer Bush Zucchini, 124
coffee can
   for sack or bag garden, 93
coffee grounds, 44
collards
   companion planting, 126, 127
   how much light, 116
   in sack garden, 94
collecting, fog, 67
college, 141
comfrey, 59
commercial farming methods, 42
common millet, 124
community gardens, 140
compacting the soil, 40, 51
companion planting, 125, 128
compost, 43, 87
   adding to the soil, 43
   as mulch, 44
   commercial         countertop
      systems, 150
   finding materials, 138
   how to make, 44
   human manure and, 48
   in grow bags, 92
   in keyhole garden, 98
   in lasagna garden, 85
   in soda bottle self-waterer, 90
   in swales, 111
   killer, 45, 135, 150
   speeding up, 45
   test for killer, 136
   toilet, 48
   toxic, 135
   tumblers, commercial, 150
compost basket, 98
compost tumbler, 46
composting
   in a nutshell, 44
composting toilets, 49
concrete

and water runoff, 59
   in spiral garden, 100
congo bean, 122
conserving water, 36
container gardening, 77
container growing
   air pruning, 133
containers
   sub-irrigated planters, 85
   toilet tanks, 136
   watering and, 77
contour lines, 108
Cook's cabbage, 122
corn
   Anasazi Sweet, 124
   and drought resistance, 122
   and the three sisters, 128
   companion planting, 127, 128
   how much light, 117
   in hugelkultur, 104
cosmos, 129
countertop compost systems, 150
cover, shade, 57
cowpeas
   and drought resistance, 122
cows, 44
cress, 115
   how much light, 116
crop rotation, 16
   in square foot garden, 84
crop variety, 38
cucumber
   Armenian, 124
   Beit Alpha, 124
   in frozen yogurt, 139
cucumbers
   companion planting, 126, 127, 128
   how much light, 117
daikon, 51, 115
   how much light, 116
dairy free ice cream book, 139
dampening off, 130

dams, 30
date, 122
David Holmgren, 37
deep planting
    and seed starting, 82
deep watering, 75
Dengue Fever, 85
denuded areas
    and runoff, 34
Department of Agriculture, 16
desert, 24, 26, 115, 119
    fog collecting in, 67
    plant adaptation, 27
    Saudi Arabia, 146
    seed starting in, 82
desert mallow, 123
detergent and graywater, 65
dill, 59, 129
    companion planting, 126, 127
    in spiral garden, 101
dinosaur kale, 124
dirt, 39
disaster, 13
diseases, 41, 130, 134, 142
    and mulch, 53
    and native plants, 114
    and perennials, 114
    balance in natural farming, 38
    Dengue Fever, 85
    encephalitis, 85
    from humanure, 49
    heartworm, 85
    malaria, 85
    transmitted by mosquitoes,
        149
    West Nile Virus, 85
dogs
    heartworm in, 85
    manure, 45
dormancy, 120
dragon fruit, 124
drainage,water, in different soil
    textures, 39

drip irrigation, 69, 147
    bottles and, 73
    in bottle tower garden, 95
drought
    Global Drought Information
        System website, 3
drought resistant fruits, 124
drought resistant herbs, 123
drought resistant other plants,
    124
drought resistant varieties, 124
drought-resistant or normal, 120
drought-tolerant versus drought-
    resistant, 119
dry farming
    and seed starting, 82
ducks, 47
    and erosion, 61
earthworms, 42, 44, 53
ecosystems, 27, 29, 40
eggplant, 130
    how much light, 117
    varieties of, 20
    Waimanalo Long, 125
encephalitis, 85
endive
    how much light, 116
engineering, water
    gabions, 111
    swales, 107
Environmental          Protection
    Agency, 14
EPA.    See    Environmental
    Protection Agency
escape route for water runoff, 59
Ethiopia, 32
evaporation, 35, 36
    factors that increase, 53
    from transpiration, 52
    preventing, in keyhole garden,
        99
    reducing, 52
fabric, 133

for fog collectors, 69
grow bags, *91*
in air pruning/sub-irrigation
  hybrids, 92
in keyhole garden, 99
in soda bottle self waterer, 91
in soda bottle self-waterer, 89
in sub-irrigated planters, 86, 88
factors needing more water, 78
fast-growing varieties, 115
fatweed, 123
faucets, 63
fence
  and reducing wind, 58
  as shade, 57
  in bottle tower garden, 95
fennel, 129
  companion planting, 126
fermenting, 138
fertilizers
  human urine as, 49
fig, 122
film
  about wood chips as mulch, 54
  Back to Eden, 54, 147
finding compost materials, 138
flies, carrot, 127
flowers
  alyssum, 129
  calendula, and drought
    resistance, 123
  California native flowers, 123
  California poppy, 123
  cosmos, 129
  desert mallow, 123
  drought resistant, 123
  Gaillardia, 123
  gladiolas, and companion
    planting, 126
  Lantana, 123
  marigolds, 129
  marigolds, companion
    planting, 126

marigolds, drought resistance,
  124
Mexican sunflowers, 123
moonflowers, 123
morning glories, 123
Osteospermum, 123
Salvias, 123
sunflowers, 129
sunflowers, and drought
  resistance, 123
sunflowers, and the three
  sisters, 128
sunflowers, companion
  planting, 126, 127, 128
Tithonia, 123
flushing a toilet
  how to flush with reused
    water, 63
fog collecting, 67
fog collectors
  how to make, 67
fog fences, 67
food poisoning, *17*
food preservation, 138
food prices, 5
food recalls, 17, 146
food safety, 14
food security, 13
food-borne illness, 17
forest, 43
  growth in, 24
forums, 142
foxtail millet, 124
free materials
  and compost, 45
free seeds, 137
free woodchips, 46
fruit trees
  and wood chips, 54
fruits
  apples, baking with, 138
  baking with, 138

dragon fruit, drought resistance, 124
drought resistant, 124
Litchi tomato, drought resistance, 124
passionfruit, drought resistance, 124
pears, baking with, 138
pitahaya, drought resistance, 124
pitaya, drought resistance, 124
pomegranate, drought resistance, 124
prickly pear, drought resistance, 124
strawberries, companion planting, 126, 127
strawberries, in ice cream, 139
strawberries, in sack garden, 94
watermelon, drought resistance, 124
watermelon, drought resistant varieties, 125
Fukuoka, Masanobu, 37
fungi, 39, 41, 42
   and hyphae, 49
   mycorrhizal, 49, 87
gabions, 111, 149
gaillardia, 123
gandul, 122
garden
   African, 146
   aquaponic, 95
   bottle tower, 95, 146
   bottle tower, how to make, 96
   fish in aquaponic, 95
   grid, 83
   herb, 99, 146
   keyhole, 97, 146
   kitchen, 8
   lasagna, 85
   pee-ponic, 95

pizza, 97
plastic bottle, 146
PVC pipe, 95
PVC pipe, how to make, 97
sack or bag, 93
soda bottle, 146
spiral, 99, 146
spiral, how to make, 100
square foot, 84
urban, 8
urine in pee-ponic, 95
Victory, 8
waffle, 83
xeriscape, 141
garden center, 141
garden paths, 51
garden types, 36, 83
gardeners
   how to find others, 140
gardening
   backyard, 24
   with children, 22
gardening myths, 148
gardening on a budget, 135
gardening tips, 134
gardening, square foot, 84
garlic
   companion planting, 126, 127, 128
gases, greenhouse, 10
Gautschi, Paul, 54, 147
Genetically Modified Organisms, 6
German millet, 124
germination, 117
   watering and, 77
germination, seed
   mulch and, 53
ghetto, 93
gladiolas
   companion planting, 126
global warming, 9, 33
GMOs, 6
goats, 29, 30, 32, 44

grains, 144
    amaranth, and drought
      resistance, 122
    millet, drought resistance, 124
    teff, drought resistance, 124
grass
    as mulch, 53
    in compost, 44
    in hugelkultur, 103
gravel
    and water runoff, 59
    in sack or bag garden, 93
    in spiral garden, 100
    in sub-irrigated planters, 88
graywater, 64
green onions
    how much light, 116
    in sack garden, 94
    in spiral garden, 101
    starting from old, 138
greenhouse
    gases, 10
    in keyhole garden, 99
greens
    collards, in sack garden, 94
    in sack or bag garden, 94
    kale, in sack garden, 94
    Swiss chard, in sack garden, 94
    turnip, 115
greywater. See graywater
grid garden, 83
ground covers, 114
groundcovers
    to slow water, 60
grow bags, 91
guandu, 122
gumbo, 122
gutter
    for rainwater collecting, 66
hardscapes
    and water runoff, 59
    escape route and, 60
harvest ideas, 138

heartworm, 85
heirloom seeds, 12, 119
herbs
    anise hyssop, 129
    arugula, in spiral garden, 101
    basil, companion planting, 125
    basil, drought resistance, 123
    basil, in ice cream, 139
    basil, in spiral garden, 101
    basil, starting another plant,
      138
    borage, 129
    chamomile, in spiral garden,
      101
    chives, companion planting,
      127
    chives, in sack garden, 94
    chives, in spiral garden, 101
    cilantro, in spiral garden, 101
    comfrey, 59
    companion planting, 126
    dill, 59, 129
    dill, companion planting, 126
    dill, in spiral garden, 101
    drought resistant, 123
    fatweed, 123
    fennel, 129
    fennel, companion planting,
      126
    hyssop, companion planting,
      126
    in spiral garden, 99, 101
    Italian parsley, 129
    lavender, 52
    lavender, drought resistance,
      123
    lavender, in spiral garden, 101
    lemon balm, in spiral garden,
      101
    lemongrass, drought
      resistance, 123
    lemongrass, in spiral garden,
      101

lemongrass, starting another plant, 138
little hogweed, 123
marjoram, in spiral garden, 101
mint, in frozen yogurt, 139
mint, in spiral garden, 101
mint, starting another plant, 138
oregano, in spiral garden, 101
parsley, companion planting, 125, 128
parsley, drought resistance, 123
parsley, in spiral garden, 101
pennyroyal, in spiral garden, 101
peppermint, companion planting, 126
pigweed, 123
purslane, 123
pursley, 123
pussley, 123
rosemary, 52
rosemary, companion planting, 126, 127
rosemary, drought resistance, 123
rosemary, in sack garden, 94
rosemary, in spiral garden, 101
sage, companion planting, 126, 127
sage, drought resistance, 123
sage, in spiral garden, 101
sorrel, drought resistance, 123
sorrel, in spiral garden, 101
spiral garden, 146
summer savory, companion planting, 126
tarragon, in spiral garden, 101
thyme, companion planting, 126
thyme, drought resistance, 123
thyme, in sack garden, 94

thyme, in spiral garden, 101
verdolaga, 123
wild portulaca, 123
wormwood, 59
wormwood, companion planting, 126, 127
yarrow, 59
hog millet, 124
Holmgren, David, 37
homegrown tomatoes, 18
homesteading, 143
Hopi, 131
horses, 44, 45
house as shade, 57
how much sunlight, 115
how much to water, 76
how often to water containers, 77
how to collect rainwater, 65
how to find other gardeners, 140
how to get seeds, 137
how to make bottle tower garden, 96
how to make compost, 44
how to make fog collectors, 67
how to make PVC pipe garden, 97
how to make sack or bag garden, 93
how to plant, 132
how to start new plants from old, 138
how to test for killer compost, 136
hugelkultur, 103
    trees to avoid, 104
human population, 9
humanure, 48
humus, 40
Hungarian millet, 124
hybrid seeds, 12
hybrids
    air pruning/sub-irrigation, 92
hyphae, 49, 50
hyssop
    companion planting, 126

ice cream, 138
ice cream book, 139
Identifying, 142
immune theory, 41
Indians
    three sisters, 128
indigenous people, 38
insects, 21, 42, 134, 142
    and companion planting, 125
    and fog collectors, 68
    balance in natural farming, 38
    **bees**, 129
    **beneficial**, 129
    carrot flies, 127
    in desert, 25
    white cabbage butterfly, 126
invasive plants, 121, 149
irrigation
    drip, from 5-gallon bucket, 147
    drip, using plastic bag, 147
irrigation, drip or trickle, 69
Italian millet, 124
jalapeno peppers
    and drought resistance, 122
Japan
    natural farming, 37
    radiation in tuna from, 11
Jimmy Nardello's Sweet Pepper,
    124
jungle, 24
kale, 21, 50, 115
    companion planting, 126
    Dinosaur or Lacinato, 124
    how much light, 116
    in sack garden, 94
    in spiral garden, 100
    Lacinato, 124
    price, 5
    Red Russian, 125
katuk, 114
kelp, 87
Kentucky Wonder Pole Bean, 124
keyhole garden, 97, 146

kiddie pools
    and sub-irrigated planters, 85
kids, 22
killer compost, 45, 135, 150
    file a report, 150
    testing for, 136
kitchen compost, 46
kitchen garden, 8
kits
    beermaking, 144
    cheesemaking, 144
    commercial        sub-irrigated
        planters, 149
    contaminated broccoli salad,
        17
    winemaking, 144
kohlrabi, 50
    companion planting, 126, 128
    how much light, 117
*kokihi*, 122
Lacinato Kale, 124
ladies' fingers, 122
landscape modification
    gabions, 111
    swales, 107
landscape, modifying, 102
lantana, 123
lasagna garden, 85
lavender, 52
    drought resistance, 123
    in spiral garden, 101
lawn mower to shred leaves, 54
layering in garden, 85
leaks, water, 62
learn more, 140
leaves
    as mulch, 53
    in hugelkultur, 103
    wilting, 76
Lebanese White Bush Marrow
    Squash, 124
leeks
    companion planting, 126, 127

leggy, 130
legumes
  peanuts, drought resistance, 124
lemon balm
  how much light, 116
  in spiral garden, 101
lemongrass
  drought resistance, 123
  in spiral garden, 101
  starting from old, 138
lettuce, 115
  companion planting, 127
  how much light, 116
  in sack garden, 94
  in square foot garden, 84
light, how much, 115
links to more information, 145
list of invasive plants, 149
Listeria, 17
litchi tomato, 124
little hogweed, 123
lizards, 21
  in desert, 25
loam, 40
local plants, 113
Loess Plateau, 29
logs in hugelkultur, 103
long beans, 122
lovegrass, 124
making compost, 44
Malabar spinach, 122
malaria, 85
manure
  cat, 45
  chicken, and wood chips, 48, 54
  dog, 45
  human, 48
  in compost, 44
Marconi Peppers, 125
marigolds, 124, 129
  companion planting, 125, 126
marjoram

in spiral garden, 101
Masanobu Fukuoka, 37
meat
  eating and global warming, 9
Mediterranean climate, 52
melon, pepino, 124
melons, 56
Mexican Sour Gherkin, 125
Mexican sunflower, 123
microbes in soil, 43
microbiology, 41
microclimates, 130
microorganisms, 41, 146
Mid-Atlantic, 145
mil ethipiene, 124
mini ecosystem, 14
mint
  how much light, 116
  in frozen yogurt, 139
  in spiral garden, 101
  starting another plant, 138
mist collecting, 67
mites, 42
mizuna, 115
modifying your landscape, 102
  gabions, 111
  swales, 107
moisture retention, 40
mold and wood chips, 47
Mollison, Bill, 37
mono-cropping, 27
moonflowers, 123
more information
  links to, 145
morning glories, 123
mosquitoes, 85, 92, 149
moth beans, 122
moths, 129
mower to shred leaves, 54
muffins, 138
mulch, 53, 128
  and slugs, 56
  and snails, 56

benefits of, 53
in hugelkultur, 104
in swales, 111
sheet, 55
using compost, 44
mustard, 50, 122
how much light, 116
mycorrhizal fungi, 49, 87
myths
gardening, debunked, 148
nasturtiums
in spiral garden, 100
Native American
three sisters, 128
Native American Indians, 131
native plants, 113
natural farming, 37
nature, 21
connection to, 18
growth in, 24
nematodes, 42, 43, 125
nets, fog, 67
New Scoop
ice cream book, 139
New Zealand spinach
and drought resistance, 122
newspaper
and worms, 48
for sheet mulching, 55
in compost, 44
in lasagna garden, 85
in soda bottle self waterer, 91
pots, 148
pots for starting seeds, 80
pots, form from PVC pipe, 148
pots, form using a can, 149
pots, making with a wine bottle, 149
pots, planting with, 132
nitrogen materials in compost, 44
nondairy ice cream book, 139
nopales, 124
nuclear radiation, 11

nurseries and garden centers, 141
nutrients, 18
Okinawan spinach, 114
okra
and drought resistance, 122
olive, 122
ollas, 71
onions
companion planting, 126, 127, 128
online resources, 142
open-pollinated seeds, 12, 119
Opuntia, 124
ordering seeds, 143
oregano
how much light, 116
in spiral garden, 101
organic
farming, regulation of, 16
regulations, 145
organic material,role in farming, 38
organic matter and soil composition, 40
osteospermum, 123
overflow
for rainwater collecting, 67
in sub-irrigated planters, 88
overhead watering, 69
paddle cactus, 124
palms, 26, 122
Panicum miliaceum, 124
paper towels
in soda bottle self waterer, 91
parsley
and drought resistance, 123
companion planting, 125, 128
how much light, 116
in spiral garden, 101
parsley, Italian, 129
parsnips
how much light, 117
passionfruit, 124

paths
  and water runoff, 59
  material to use to prevent
    runoff, 59
paths, garden, 51
pathway
  in swales, 111
Paul Gautschi, 54, 147
peanuts, 124
pears
  in muffins and cakes, 138
peas
  companion planting, 128
  companion planting, 127, 128
  eating from the garden, 18
  how much light, 117
  in hugelkultur, 104
peat moss, 43
peat-moss, 86
pee-ponics, 95
pennyroyal
  in spiral garden, 101
pepino, 124
peppermint
  companion planting, 126
peppers, 56, 130, 132
  and drought resistance, 122
  how much light, 117
  Jimmy Nardello's Sweet, 124
  Marconi, 125
  Thai chili, 125
  varieties of, 20
perennials, 114
permaculture, 37, 143
  gabions, 149
  hugelkultur, 103
  video, 150
Perpetual Spinach Chard, 125
pest control, 134
pesticides
  and killer compost, 45
  definition of, 15
  tolerances, 15

pests, 134
  and native plants, 114
  and perennials, 114
  balance in natural farming, 38
  carrot flies, 127
  in wood chips, 47
  white cabbage butterflies, 126
Pests, 142
photosynthesis, 39, 43, 52
pickling, 138
pigeon peas, 122
pigweed, 123
Pinky Popcorn, 125
pipe
  for graywater, 64
pipes
  long, for irrigation, 74
pitahaya, 124
pitaya, 124
pizza garden, 97
plant
  starting from old, 138
planter
  sub-irrigated, 149
planters
  toilet tanks, 136
planting, 113
  companion, 125
  for square foot garden, 84
  how to plant, 132
  when to plant, 131
  where to plant, 130
planting deeply
  seed starting and, 82
planting seeds, 117
planting, companion, 128
  three sisters, 128
plants
  for providing shade, 57
  in spiral garden, 100, 101
  invasive, 149
  native, 113

that attract beneficial
  insects, 129
**that attract pollinators**, 129
to reduce wind, 58
watering, 69
plants that tolerate heat and
  drought well, 122
plastic
  bottle self-waterer, 89
  bottle tower garden, 95
plastic bag, 147
plastic bags
  sack or bag garden, 93
plastic bottles, 146
plastic sheeting
  as sheet mulch, 56
  in keyhole garden, 99
plumb bob, 109
poisoned
  compost, 45
pole
  in bottle tower garden, 95
pole beans
  companion planting, 126, 127
**pollinating insects and bugs**,
  129
pomegranate, 124
popcorn
  Pinky, 125
population, 9
potatoes
  companion planting, 126, 127,
    128
pots
  air pruning, 133
  air pruning/sub-irrigation, 92
  broken, in spiral garden, 100
  newspaper, form from PVC
    pipe, 148
  newspaper, making from a can,
    149
  newspaper, making with a
    wine bottle, 149

potting mix, 40
potting soil, 86
poultry manure in compost, 44
prepping, 13
prices
  food, 5
  for seeds, 5
  kale, 5
prickly pear, 124
proso millet, 124
protozoa, 42
pruning, air, 92, 133, 150
pumpkin
  and drought resistance, 122
  and the three sisters, 128
  companion planting, 127, 128
  how much light, 117
  in muffins and cakes, 138
purslane, 123
pursley, 123
pussley, 123
PVC garden
  how to make, 97
PVC pipe
  for making newspaper pots, 82
  for sack garden, 93
  garden, 95
  garden, how to make, 97
rabbits, 44
radiation
  in tuna from Japan, 11
radishes, 115
  companion planting, 127
  how much light, 117
rain
  barrels, 147
rain gutter, 149
rain gutters
  and sub-irrigated planters, 85
rainforest, 26
rainwater, 147
  collecting, 65
  how to collect, 65

rainwater collecting
  chain, 66
  gutter and, 66
  overflow for, 67
rainwater collection
  in China, 30
  in Saudi Arabia, 31
Rattlesnake Pole Bean, 125
real world, 29
recalls, 17, 145
recycling, 25
red gram, 122
Red Russian Kale, 125
reducing wind, 58
resources, 140
respect for what you grow, 19
retaining moisture in soil with
  organic matter, 40
rhubarb, 114, 124
rocks
  as mulch, 56
  in keyhole garden, 98
  in sack gardens, 93
  in soil composition, 39
  in spiral garden, 100
  next to trees, 56
  walls, 149
root vegetables
  and soil compaction, 51
root-bound
  seedlings, 119
roots
  air pruning, 92, 133
  air-pruning, 150
  development, 149
rosemary, 52
  companion planting, 126, 127
  drought resistance, 123
  in sack garden, 94
  in spiral garden, 101
rotation, crop, 16
rotifers, 42
runoff, 14, 34, 35, 36

reducing, 52, 59
slowing with organic material,
  60
rutabega
  how much light, 117
rutabegas
  companion planting, 126
safety, food, 14
sage
  companion planting, 126, 127
  drought resistance, 123
  in spiral garden, 101
salt tolerant vegetables, 122
salvias, 123
sandy soil, 39
Saudi Arabia, 31, 146
saving seeds, 11, 137, 145
sawdust
  in swales, 111
scallions
  how much light, 116
scarification, 118
schools, gardening in, 22
sea spinach, 122
seasonal eating, 20
seasons,eating with the, 20
seed saving, 145
seed starting
  dry farming and, 82
seedlings, 118
  tips for peppers and tomatoes,
  132
seedlings tips, 130
seeds
  and germination by birds, 27
  free, 137
  germination and watering, 77
  grains, 144
  heirloom, 12, 119
  how to get, 137
  hybrid, 12
  in hugelkultur, 104
  open-pollinated, 12, 119

paper towel and starting, 78
planting, 117
prices, 5
saving, 11, 137
scarification, 118
sources for, 143
starting, 78
starting indoors, 118
storing, 138
tray for starting, 79
self watering
soda bottles, 89
self watering tray for starting seeds, 79
self-watering
beds and containers, 88
*Setaria italica*, 124
shade
in keyhole garden, 99
shade cloth
for shade cover, 57
shade cloths, 78
shade, building a, 57
shade, providing, 57
shallots
companion planting, 128
sheep, 44
sheet mulch
using plastic sheeting, 56
sheet mulching, 55
shower heads, 63
showering
conserving water while, 63
shrubs, 114
to slow water, 60
silt, 39
SIPs. *See* sub-irrigated planters
slowing runoff, 60
slugs, 42, 134
and mulch, 56
in grow bags, 92
small varieties, 115
snails, 42

and mulch, 56
soap and graywater, 65
sod
in hugelkultur, 104
soda bottles, 146
in tower garden, 95
self waterers, 89
soil
role of, 39
soil microbes, 43
Soil structure and composition, 39
sorrel
drought resistance, 123
in spiral garden, 101
soups, 138
sources for seeds, 143
Southeastern, 145
Southwest, 144
space when planting
for square foot garden, 84
spiders
in desert, 25
spinach, 50
how much light, 116
in muffins and cakes, 138
Okinawan, 114
Perpetual Spinach Chard, 125
spinach, New Zealand
and drought resistance, 122
spiral garden, 99, 146
springtails, 42
square foot garden
and crop rotation, 84
square foot gardening, 84
squash, 115
and the three sisters, 128
companion planting, 127
how much light, 117
large, 21
Lebanese White Bush Marrow, 124
starting new green onions from old, 138

starting new plants from old, 138
starting seeds
    in paper towels, 78
    in tray, 79
    newspaper pots for, 80
starting seeds indoors, 118
sticks
    in keyhole garden, 98
stones
    in keyhole garden, 98
storing seeds, 138
straw
    in hugelkultur, 103
    in keyhole garden, 98
    in swales, 111
strawberries
    companion planting, 126, 127
    eating from the garden, 18
    how much light, 117
    in ice cream, 139
    in sack garden, 94
sub-irrigated
    5-gallon bucket planters, 150
    grow bags, 91
    planter kits, 149
    planter using organic
        materials, 149
    self-watering bottles, 89
sub-irrigated planter
    grow bags, 91
sub-irrigated planters, 85
    and kiddie pools, 85
    and rain gutters, 85
    buckets and, 86
    overflow hole, 88
sub-irrigation, 74
    rain gutter system, 149
succulents, 27, 119
succulents and compost, 44
Sugar Baby Watermelon, 125
summer savory
    companion planting, 126
sunflower

Mexican, 123
sunflowers, 22, 129
    and drought resistance, 123
    and the three sisters, 128
    companion planting, 126, 127,
        128
    in hugelkultur, 104
sustainable, 7
swales, 107
sweet pepino, 124
sweet potato
    and drought resistance, 122
    in ice cream, 139
Swiss chard
    and drought resistance, 123
    how much light, 116
    in sack garden, 94
    Perpetual Spinach, 125
symbiotic relationships, 27
taf, 124
tarragon
    in spiral garden, 101
teas, 138
teff, 124
telephone books in keyhole
    garden, 98
tepary beans, 144
    and drought resistance, 123
terra cotta
    ollas, 71
terra cotta pots
    as ollas, 73
    in keyhole garden, 98
terracing, 30, 31
testing for killer compost, 136
tetragon, 122
Thai Chili Peppers, 125
theory of immunity, 41
three sisters, 128
thyme
    and drought resistance, 123
    companion planting, 126
    in sack garden, 94

in spiral garden, 101
tilling, 50
tilling the soil, 42
tips
    gardening on a budget, 135
    general gardening, 134
tips for healthy seedlings, 130
tips for pepper and tomato
    seedlings, 132
Tithonia, 123
toilet
    flushing, 62
    flushing and wasting water, 63
    flushing with reused water, 63
**toilet tanks**, 136
toilets, composting, 49
tolerances, 15
tomatoes, 56, 130, 132
    and drought resistance, 123
    Arkansas Traveler, 124
    companion planting, 125
    how much light, 117
    in hugelkultur, 104
    in muffins and cakes, 138
    in square foot garden, 84
    taste of homegrown versus
        store-bought, 18
    varieties of, 20
toothbrushing, 62
toxic, 104
transpiration, 35, 52, 58
transplanting
    watering and, 77
transportation, 18
traps, fog, 67
tray for starting seeds, 79
tree mulch, 46
tree trimmers
    getting wood chips from, 47
tree trimming services
    getting wood chips from, 47
trees, 30, 114
    and rocks, 56

as shade, 57
drought tolerant, 122
in hugelkultur, 103
in swales, 111
to reduce wind, 58
to slow water, 60
trees to avoid
    in hugelkultur, 104
trickle irrigation, 69
tumblers, Compost, 150
turnips, 50, 113
    companion planting, 126, 128
    greens, 115
    how much light, 117
types of gardens, 36, 83
university extension offices, 141
unusual ice cream flavors, 139
urban garden, 8
urine
    human, 48
    human, as plant spray, 49
    in hugelkultur, 103
USDA, 16
using A-frame tool, 110
using toilet tanks as planters, 136
varieties
    drought-resistant, 124
    of carrots, 20
    of eggplant, 20
    of lettuce, 20
    of peppers, 20
    of tomatoes, 20
variety of crops, 38
vegan ice cream book, 139
vegetables
    amaranth, and drought
        resistance, 122
    asparagus beans, and drought
        resistance, 122
    asparagus, and drought
        resistance, 122
    asparagus, companion
        planting, 125, 128

baking with, 138
bamia, 122
beans, and drought resistance, 122
beans, and the three sisters, 128
beans, companion planting, 126
beans, drought resistant varieties, 124, 125
beets, companion planting, 126
bhindi, 122
black-eyed peas, and drought resistance, 122
Botany Bay spinach, 122
broccoli, companion planting, 126
Brussels sprouts, companion planting, 126
bush beans, companion planting, 126
bush beans,companion planting, 126
cabbage family, companion planting, 126
cabbage, companion planting, 126, 127, 128
carrots, baking with, 138
carrots, companion planting, 126
cauliflower, companion planting, 126
celery, companion planting, 127
chili peppers, drought resistant varieties, 125
chives, companion planting, 126, 127
collards, companion planting, 126, 127
congo beans, 122
Cook's cabbage, 122

corn, and drought resistance, 122
corn, and the three sisters, 128
corn, companion planting, 127, 128
corn, drought resistant varieties, 124
cowpeas, and drought resistance, 122
cucumber, drought resistant varieties, 124
cucumber, in frozen yogurt, 139
cucumbers, companion planting, 126, 127, 128
drought resistant, 122
eggplant, drought resistant varieties, 125
eggplants, 130
gandul, 122
garlic, companion planting, 126, 127, 128
green onions, starting from old, 138
guandu, 122
gumbo, 122
jalapenos, and drought resistance, 122
kale, companion planting, 126
kale, drought resistant varieties, 124, 125
kohlrabi, companion planting, 126, 128
kokihi, 122
ladies' fingers, 122
leeks, companion planting, 126, 127
lettuce, companion planting, 127
long beans, and drought resistance, 122
Malabar spinach, 122
moth beans, 122

mustard, and drought resistance, 122

New Zealand spinach, and drought resistance, 122

nopales, drought resistance, 124

okra, and drought resistance, 122

onions, companion planting, 126, 127, 128

peas, companion planting, 127, 128

pepino melon, drought resistance, 124

pepino, drought resistance, 124

peppers, 130, 132

peppers, and drought resistance, 122

peppers, drought resistant varieties, 124

pigeon peas, 122

pole beans, and companion planting, 126

pole beans, companion planting, 126, 127

popcorn, drought resistant varieties, 125

potatoes, companion planting, 126, 127, 128

pumpkin, and the three sisters, 128

pumpkin, baking with, 138

pumpkin, companion planting, 127, 128

pumpkins, and drought resistance, 122

radishes, companion planting, 127

red gram, 122

rhubarb, drought resistance, 124

rutabegas, companion planting, 126

salt tolerant, 122

sea spinach, 122

shallots, companion planting, 128

spinach, baking with, 138

spinach, drought resistant varieties, 125

squash, and the three sisters, 128

squash, companion planting, 127

squash, drought resistant varieties, 124

sweet pepino, drought resistance, 124

sweet potato, and drought resistance, 122

sweet potato, in ice cream, 139

Swiss chard, and drought resistance, 122

Swiss chard, drought resistant varieties, 125

tepary beans, and drought resistance, 122

tetragon, 122

tomatoes, 130, 132

tomatoes, and drought resistance, 122

tomatoes, baking with, 138

tomatoes, companion planting, 125

tomatoes, drought resistant varieties, 124

turnips, companion planting, 126, 128

Warrigal greens, 122

yard long beans, and drought resistance, 122

zucchini, baking with, 138

zucchini, drought resistant varieties, 124

verdolaga, 123
vermiculture, 48
vertical gardening, 146
   bottle tower garden, 95
Victory Gardens, 8
video
   bacteria, 146
   permaculture, 150
vinegar, 138
vines
   for shade, 57
waffle garden, 83
Waimanalo Long Eggplant, 125
walk to learn more, 140
wall
   in bottle tower garden, 95
walnut
   in hugelkultur, 104
warm climate varieties, 115
warming
   global, 9
Warrigal cabbage, 122
Warrigal greens, 122
washing
   reusing water, 64
water
   runoff, 14
water bottles
   in tower garden, 95
water conservation, 36, 62
water engineering, 105
   gabions, 111
   swales, 107
water runoff
   and hard surfaces, 59
   and paths, 59
   escape route for, 59
   reducing, 59
   slowing with plants, 60
watering, 36
   containers and, 77
   deeply, 75
   factors that increase, 78

   germination and, 77
   how much to, 76
   transplanting and, 77
   when to, 75
   wilting leaves and, 76
watering plants, 69
watering wand, 74
watermelon, 124
   Sugar Baby, 125
weather
   and native plants, 113
   crazy, 10
websites
   Global Drought Information System, 3
weed
   purslane, 123
weed whacker to shred leaves for mulch, 54
weeds
   balance in natural farming, 38
West Nile Virus, 85
what to do with your harvest, 138
what to grow, 113
what to plant, 113
when to plant, 131
when to water your plants, 75
where to buy seeds, 143
where to plant, 130
white millet, 124
wild portulaca, 123
wind, reducing, 58
windbreaks, 58, 78
wine, 138
   bottles in keyhole garden, 98
wine bottle
   for making newspaper pots, 82
   to make newspaper pots, 149
winemaking kits, 144
wood
   in hugelkultur, 103
wood chips, 46, 147
   and fruit trees, 54

and water runoff, 59
as mulch, 53
film, 147
film about mulch, 54
how to use them as mulch, 54
in spiral garden, 100
wood shavings, 44
wood turning
  to make newspaper pot form,
    82
woods, 24
woodturning, 105
  newspaper pots, 148
woodworking, 105

worm tea, 48
worms, 42
  and composting, 48
  and vermiculture, 48
  castings, 48
wormwood, 59
  companion planting, 126, 127
xeriscape garden, 141
yard-long beans, 122
yarrow, 59
zucchini
  Cocozelle Summer Bush, 124
  in muffins and cakes, 138

# Can you help me?

Did you like this book? Did you find it helpful? I certainly hope so.

If you did, would you consider leaving a review to let me and others know? Just a few words about what you found helpful are fine. Please visit the book's sales page on **amazon.com** and leave your review there.

If you didn't like this book or didn't find it helpful, I'd still like to hear from you. It helps me to write better books and improve as an author/illustrator.

If you need help finding some information, and there is nothing in the **References** section that will help, email me. I may be able to send you a link to more information, or otherwise answer your question.

Please email me at 4alina@alinaspencil.com

Thank you for your feedback!

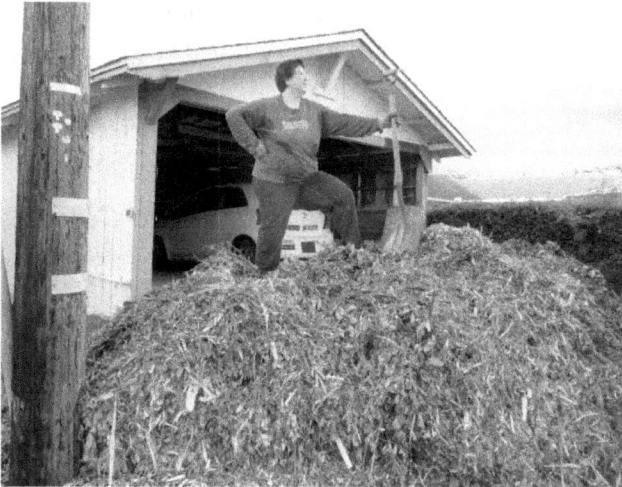

Wood chips...not for the faint of heart!

# Also by the author:

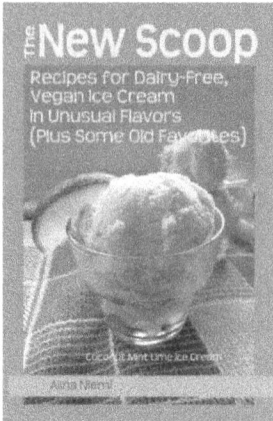

## Strange Ice Cream Flavors

Use your fruits and vegetables to make unusual flavors of ice cream, frozen yogurt, sorbet, and sherbet.

All are dairy free and delicious. Perfect if you have allergies, excess produce, or an adventurous spirit!

Includes directions for making your own mochi ice cream. Try Peanut Butter and Jelly Ice Cream.

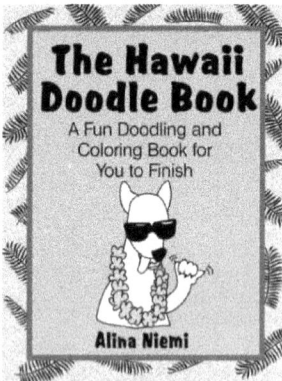

## Learn About Hawaii And Draw

Kids (and adults) of all ages can learn about Hawaii's plants, animals, food, and culture. Includes a Hawaiian language pronunciation guide and glossary.

Includes how-to-draw tips! Ages 6+

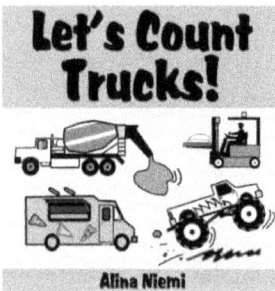

## Truck Lovers, Learn to Count!

Most children can say their numbers but get confused when using them. Help your preschool or toddler child learn to count by pointing to the colorful trucks.

Part of the **Let's Count!** Series.

www.ingramcontent.com/pod-product-compliance
Lightning Source LLC
Chambersburg PA
CBHW072004090426
42740CB00011B/2087